T0209624

43 YEAR OLD FEMALE

Diane Mullen

authorHOUSE®

AuthorHouse™
1663 Liberty Drive
Bloomington, IN 47403
www.authorhouse.com
Phone: 1 (800) 839-8640

This book is not designed to substitute for professional medical advice. The publisher and the author disclaim liability for any medical outcomes that may occur as a result of applying the methods suggested in this book.

Published by AuthorHouse   11/27/2019

ISBN: 978-1-7283-3444-8 (sc)
ISBN: 978-1-7283-3506-3 (hc)
ISBN: 978-1-7283-3443-1 (e)

Library of Congress Control Number: 2019917993

Print information available on the last page.

This book is printed on acid-free paper.

Dedication

In loving memory of my Mom and to my wonderful Dad

And…

A massive thank you to Paulo Coelho, for writing *The Alchemist.*
And to my mom, for leaving it on my pillow 25 years ago.

Acknowledgements

A special thank you to my Mom and Dad, for always believing in me. Thank you to my brother and family for the laptop in my time of need. Thank you to my good friends over the years who have kept up with me, despite my nomadic lifestyle and spontaneous nature. Thank you Lori (and your entire family), for housing me in my times of non-structure and chaos. Thank you, Kari, for keeping me sane over the last few years (and reminding me to hydrate while writing all of this)! And thanks to Ariela Wilcox, of The Wilcox Agency, for her many hours of work, support, and for tech-battling my...anything-tech-doesn't-work-around-me force field. Lastly, a big thank you to Carlsbad, CA and all the people here who have welcomed me to my new home (you know who you are).

Contents

Introduction

Let's start from the beginning. I was born in Auburn, AL in December of 1975. My dad was from upstate NY and my mom from Boston area. My brother, 2 years older, was born in NY. The 3 of them moved to Auburn several months before I was born, based on a University position for my dad (and once able, a University position for my mom as well). So, I grew up in a college town, with friends who's parents were mostly transplants as well. As a family, we made regular trips up the east coast for holidays and summer road trips to other parts of the country. These were not 'fancy' trips…I recall mostly low-end motels and a lot of time in our station wagon, which was highly air-conditioned challenged. I feel extremely lucky to have been able to travel at a young age, and my love of travel started very early and continued to grow throughout my life.

I had two very loving parents and an incredibly nice older brother. Again, I was very lucky in so many ways in terms of my childhood. At a young age, I discovered self-discipline for both schoolwork and in playing sports. I remember realizing a few things about myself very young. I never slept during nap time in Kindergarten (but it was my favorite part of the school day other than recess), because I could just lie there and relax and think about whatever I wanted to, without noise. I also would look around and be amazed that kids were actually able to sleep. I would later discover at sleep-overs as I got older that no one else would be awake most of the night like me. I wondered why, but it never struck me to ask anyone. In second grade, I found it was very easy to 'win' every coloring contest just by attention to shading and staying within the lines. These seemed like very easy things to do and natural for me, but it struck me that it was definitely NOT that way for most. I wondered why. If someone gave me something to do, I focused and completed it with the reward internally being I could then have time to do or think about what I wanted to. The reward was not so much completing it quickly and feeling efficient, it was so that I could then relax and have 'me' time. This has never changed. I always wanted 'me' time, to use and think how I wanted, to be creative in my mind as opposed to following directions. However, I was very good at following directions, paying attention to detail, and being efficient all so I could be 'free.' My other reason was strictly an energy-saver. I always felt like I was going to run out of energy (later the cause of this was obvious with an undiagnosed sleep disorder of sorts), but as long as I can remember I have been exhausted every day and just wanted to get things done in case I hit my 'wall.'

I developed techniques, without even realizing it, in the years that followed to cope with exhaustion, while still being productive. I started using the power of habit quite early. Study habits, mentally powering down to conserve energy in-between, and using exercise, nature, music, anything to give me bursts of energy. I didn't realize how much I relied on these things until years later in school, but I remember being surprised to find out when I graduated high school that I had never made anything other than A's my whole life. This was not fully on my radar until graduating.

I went on to Purdue University for my undergraduate degree in Biology, with a minor in Psychology. First, I realized just how tough decisions were for me while narrowing down colleges and deciding on Purdue. Once I decide something, I make sure it happens. But, initial decisions... wow, torturous! I had this strong sense about how much different my path in life would be, depending on which school I went to. Part of me knew this was true, but at the same time, no path was right or wrong. Yet, I ended up waiting until the last possible day to decide. I remember my mom standing in my doorway, checking on me to see if I had come to a conclusion. I have to say, my parents were amazing at not pushing me when they knew pushing would only make it worse. I always end up going with my gut. I just have to wade through all the practical/logical/pros and cons first, but in the end it was a gut decision. I didn't connect to it until that day. But, the feeling once I do connect, is unmistakable and intense. This has happened many times over my life, but only when I am able/allow myself to be in tune with my inner voice. It's there, it just gets drowned out with all the noise around me.

While at Purdue, I had a guidance counselor who was concerned about my indecision about how I wanted to use my biology degree (and what, out of interest, ended up including a psychology minor). She gave me a test of some kind that was supposed to let you know where your 'job' interests may be if you were having trouble picturing yourself in any particular type of job. My 'interest level' score was 7%. This did not surprise me one bit, but um, apparently this was the lowest score anyone had scored in the 25+ years she was counseling. She seemed quite distraught. The funny part to me was that the results said that I should either be a firefighter or a flower arranger. Although it was hilarious to me at the time, later, I thought maybe it wasn't too far off. I basically had trained myself to run off of adrenaline and I had a strong sense I wanted to find a way to bring happiness into people's lives if I could. So, part-time firefighter and part-time flower arranger could have worked!

As was my way, I decided as late as possible, based on a gut decision, to become a Physical Therapist. I had dealt with injuries of my own since I was a kid and had experience in physical therapy leading up to graduating (including a knee surgery right before my senior year), as well as having to deal with my own mental adaptation of not being able to do what I loved (sports) and finding ways to enjoy what I could.

Since I did not come to this conclusion until late in college, this meant my last year in college was packed with all the requirements to get into PT school. During this time, I got mono, had an extreme reaction to a medication I was given to combat nausea, ended up in the ER, and missed finals. Once stabilized from the reaction, I had to then fight through mono-fatigue as well as my own baseline fatigue and miss the spring break week to make up finals. I will say, I had to harness all my energy-habits to get through and into PT school at Washington University in St. Louis. And, that was the easy part.

My battle continued throughout grad school in that I was exhausted, was in the most rigorous PT program in the country at the time, had several illnesses that 1) never fit any diagnosis and 2) my body always reacted to any medication given. In short, my body did not respond in the ways expected, for most any condition/illness that I experienced. This included another 'condition' that I had been dealing with for many years, which was an undiagnosed condition where my body would decide to pass out. The first episode was in 7th grade in the school lunch line. Through the years I had many tests and doctors, but it did not fit any diagnosis. It seemed to be 'random,' but over the years I learned to constantly self-monitor the symptoms and adapt to avoid fully losing consciousness (most of the time). I also figured out an exercise regimen to gradually increase my threshold of activity (for the part that was activity-dependent) to increase the intensity it took to create symptoms. I started figuring this out in my 20s and still use it today to keep my body at its highest possible fully-conscious state! Everything depended on consistency, attention to detail, and subtle modifications in what I was doing, with careful progression. I had to train my mind to monitor symptoms and train my body to withstand increased activity.

After graduating PT school, I spent the next 17 years treating patients with all kinds of injuries and pain conditions. I used what I knew from school, as well as all I had learned over the years treating myself (with the attention to detail that I had given myself, because every body responds differently to injury/healing and every mind needs training to make new habits and modifications). I applied the same idea of gradually increasing the threshold that the body would 'react' negatively, staying just below the onset of increased inflammation/over-treatment in order to heal as efficiently and progressively as possible. The other piece I incorporated was to address how difficult it was for people to follow a home exercise program by making sure the programs were step-wise and clear. I developed a plan for patients to get them to do a couple exercises exactly right and schedule those exercises into their daily routine (habit training), and then to build on that without overwhelming either them or their body. The idea being to establish a foundation (both body and habit), increase it but below the threshold of losing ground, consistency and repetition for the body and habits to adjust, and persistent progress that was sustainable.

Overall, I knew I was doing good things for a lot of people and enjoyed that part, but I had a nagging feeling that I was going to hit a point where I would no longer be able to fit my need for 'me' time, time to travel, feed my soul, and bust out of what was a down-to-every-single-minute style of work that was burning me out both mentally and physically. Given my energy/sleep challenge every day, coupled with an intense carpe diem/life-is-short attitude towards life, I was getting antsy in a way that was growing quickly. I always had this feeling of 'live it now' (possibly due to a feeling like I might one day hit my ultimate energy expenditure wall and be … well, life-spent) and tried to incorporate as much of my 'needs' as possible into a very structured job/career. I did travel PT for 7 of the17 years of working as a physical therapist, moving every 3 months (or staying in 3-month chunks if I wanted) in order to travel the U.S. and work full time at the same time, while allowing for travel between contracts. That helped, but it was an intense way to live and was a life of constant change. I knew eventually I would need a home-base and I felt very early on it would end up being

CA. I can remember longing to be in CA as a young kid, before I had ever been there or even knew why.

A few things about me, which maybe are obvious to you already. I had a hard time with decisions. But once I decided something, BLAM. It was happening. Not immediately (although that was sometimes the case), but I knew it was not worth fighting - it was GOING to happen, so I might as well get on board! This ties into the whole go-after-your-bucket-list-as-if-you-may-kick-the-bucket-any-day attitude... which, well, is the case for all of us since we all are in the category of having a finite number of days in our life and we don't know how many. I was not into the idea of waiting until the 'perfect' time for a trip or waiting for retirement. And the more I treated people with sometimes life-altering injuries, who all came to this realization later than they wished once there was a shot of perspective, I'm sure that added to it. I always had the internal battle between my carpe diem side and my practical side. We all do on some level. But mine started kind of early... I saved every dollar I earned, starting with the first (I still have it), which was in 1984 raking leaves for neighbors. I saved as much as I could as long as I could and this habit continued throughout all my jobs... with a specific fund-my-bucket-list attitude.

I managed to travel the world and save for what would eventually be a major life-change situation, which I think I always knew would come at some point. This happened eventually in full-force at age 41. But I will get to that part in a bit. First, tragedy in my life personally. My mom was diagnosed with brain cancer in 2009 and lived 15 months. She died at 65. She was teaching and running a lab at Auburn University and one day could not get her key to open her office door. From that day onward, it was a tough battle and pure agony for me watching her decline. I left my job (at the time in WA) when she was diagnosed and prognosis was grim. I moved home to be with her and my dad during this time. I am so grateful I did have time with her, albeit a painful time. She was the most patient and loving person I have ever known. She was also the strongest. Until the end. I learned a lot about my mom, my dad, and myself during this time. My dad was the most amazingly strong and caring person throughout it all. And I learned I wasn't as strong as I thought or wanted to be. All good insights. And very hard.

After she passed, I had a long stint of full-blown insomnia and struggled with an insanely strong feeling of being lost. I realized I needed to go somewhere and that place was Italy. This was a place she and I had talked about going. She never got to go, but I wanted to go 'for her' and in a way 'with' her. Something told me that I could find a way to heal there and somehow 'get right.'

It feels a little weird to include all this personal pain in a book like this, but I cannot deny that this was a huge part of my journey to where I am today. So, once I was in Italy, I went to wine country to be in the rolling hills and sunshine and away from most people (but with excellent wine, of course, and in a region very high on my bucket list). At one point, I ended up on a walk on no particular road or trail, just walked and walked through the country-side. I came upon a massive, beautiful tree in the middle of rolling hills. And, I saw my mom in that tree. I cannot explain it more than that, but I knew that this is was why I was here. I sat down at the base of the tree and cried out everything that was so stuck inside of me. It must have been hours, but I had no sense of time. After that, I got up and from that point on, I knew I would: 1) be ok 2) make sure I was always pursuing my dreams, not getting stuck in a life that didn't at least move in that direction actively.

Upon return, I did a job search that included non-negotiable conditions on my part: 1) I would not be working a schedule that was 'expected' in the medical appointment-based world 2) I would be taking way more than 2 weeks of vacation a year 3) If I was still working for them in 2 years, I would be taking a 2-3 month leave to go to World Cup in Brazil and travel South America. Now, you might think this was extreme, but it was the only way to attempt to stay in my profession and actually MAKE those things happen. I had to risk all the 'no's until the right person agreed. Funny thing, my first choice said yes! That was the next lesson: If you don't ask, you won't get!

And now, we get to the why-I-am-telling-you-all-this-stuff part. Yes, more! Something happened once I was in my 40s. It was a convergence of a physical injury that put me out of work (with no pay) and a very tough (for me) time period of having to ask for help due to living alone and having very little use of my upper extremities; an inability to take pain meds to survive the worst part; and an escalation of my previous conditions of sleep deprivation and passing out-ness, along with a growing feeling of being trapped in a medical system/job that didn't quite fit me + full-on LIFE IS SHORT and you must stop and figure out what's next. I had a strong feeling of needing clarity, self-assessment and a rest-of-my-life trajectory check. All at once. I quit my job, put all my belongings in storage in VERY good friends' attics and extra rooms, and left the country for an undetermined period of time. I returned to the US about a month and half later and knew I needed to do a complete overhaul of my health, my mind, and my direction. I needed to tune into that same 'gut' that I had been trying to listen to since I was a kid. To do this, I knew I needed to get off the one sleep-aide that I had been using for many years to survive my work schedule. I had a feeling, even though it was how I got through life for a while and it was non-prescription and as far as anyone knew, non habit-forming, I had a feeling it was making me brain-foggy and I needed full clarity.

The next 6 months involved a process of my body slowly (very slowly) adjusting to first no sleep at all, then to a few hours, and eventually starting to be able to use my brain in any functional way again. Once I could think clearly, or mostly, I began the active search for where I wanted to live (unrelated to a job, person, or any 'normal' reasons you pick a place). I packed my car in Seattle and started down the coast to CA. I made a promise to myself that if a place 'grabbed' me immediately and forcefully in my insides, that is where I would fully recover and start my new chapter. It happened exactly that way. The place was/is Carlsbad, CA. I found a small apartment that had all my requirements: walkable to the beach, walkable to 'town,' enough space for my exercise/health routine, space for my drum kit, and a balcony with sunshine. It is tiny and the cheapest scenario around, but it is perfect. And it is where I am writing this now!

My next task was to take head-on all my health problems. I set out re-researching all my issues, experimenting on myself using exercise, diet changes/adjustments, finding a supplement that fantastically and shockingly reduced my passing out-ness along with reduced inflammation and increased energy, revamping my daily habits with regards to sleep, food, thought patterns, and finally getting to a point that I felt the most healthy and most stable I had ever remembered feeling. My brain was clear, my body was fit, and I was putting in place all the things I knew I wanted to prioritize for my own health and well-being for the years to follow.

I then started a business, focusing on helping people revamp their fitness routines and activity goals, along with trying to find a way to teach people preventative measures that I had learned over the years for better baseline body health/wellness. Since then, I realized I had even more to give/share. This has morphed into a desire to help people just like me (maybe without all the weird health conditions!) transform their lives in their 40s. There is something special about this decade. You have learned more about who you really are, what you really want, and have the desire to jumpstart the rest of your life by taking a look at where you are, what you are doing, and where you want to go. My hope in writing this book is to give you a starting point for creating a new foundation in your 40s, to serve you and assist you for the rest of your life. I truly believe this is the perfect time to re-evaluate, re-align, and re-boot your life by learning how to train your mind and body to work for you, instead of against you, towards what makes you happy and what allows you a sturdy base to support you throughout the journey ahead. We have one brain, one body, and one life. I want to help you make the most of all 3! I sincerely hope my journey and my tips/tools can help everyone who reads it, in ways big and/or small. It's not rocket-science, it's just my method.

And if there is a chance it could help any of you, too, it is worth all the work of sharing it with you.

Additionally, I have a special place in my heart for a particular subset of those of us in our 40s. I am creating unique programs and retreats for women in their 40s, who are unmarried and kid-free. I happen to be in this group at this point in my life and I feel I can especially help and relate to these women and their particular challenges, health/fitness goals, and life re-boots!

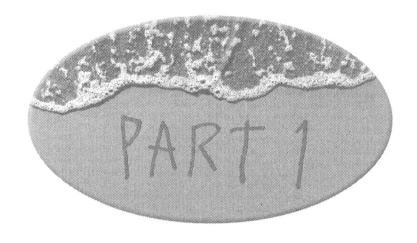

The Brain: Get Clear

CHAPTER 1

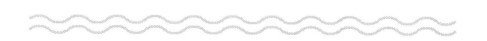

Just Stop

Let's start with the good news! If you are reading this, you have a functioning brain. Let's use it to your advantage. Think of your brain as your personal computer that only you get to program. And (unless you are like me and computers and phones and GPS and anything-tech goes berserk around you!) this is quite helpful because you can program your brain to assist you in what you want to achieve, even in your subconscious. In fact, get this, your subconscious is in charge of about 95% of information coming into your brain. This floored me when I first learned it! This means that our underlying thought patterns/beliefs, which rule our subconscious… which in turn drives our habits, are key to change in our lives.

To just throw it out there right now before we even dive deeper into the brain, we first need to reprogram our subconscious beliefs (what we really think about ourselves, what we can accomplish, how we feel about the world around us, etc.) in order to let our brain be our assistant instead of our invisible foe. If not, our results (what we want but keep failing or have trouble achieving) stay the same, even if our conscious mind desires a different result i.e. we REALLY want it. Put simply, if you have running subconscious thought patterns that say 'I can't lose weight' or 'I can lose weight, but I can't keep it off or 'I just don't have the time' or 'I don't deserve this thing' or whatever it might be… well then, the result will stay the same. We will get more into this later, but I wanted to get it out there to you so you can let it settle in a bit. This becomes extremely helpful when it comes to habit change.

For now, let's focus on the part about it being YOUR brain and only YOU can truly direct it. You are in charge of your own thought patterns, what you choose to do with information you receive, and whether you use your brain and subconscious to assist you in what you want or let it hinder you. No one likes to not have control of their own thoughts or actions, so this is great news.

Next order of business... I want to congratulate all of you that have made it to your 40s!! Whew! A wild ride I am sure. At least for most of us, when you consider all the things that have happened in your life over 40+ years that could have thwarted this achievement! So, we should first celebrate our survival to get us to this point in our lives. Let's sum up so far: you have a functioning brain AND you have successfully used it to survive (and hopefully thrive) in the process. Excellent job! Gratitude is essential for happiness in life and this is truly something to be grateful for.

Speaking of making it to your 40s (for those of you reading that are not here yet, welcome to the club eventually!), there are things that start to happen around this time that, well, can add to our challenges in life. But, I am here to try to help you navigate through these things with knowledge of good habit strategies, ways to prevent some common injuries that tend to start showing their faces more often, and tools to modify your routines during unexpected obstacles so that you can maintain all the good routines you have worked to achieve. I want to provide you with a good foundation of both body and brain habits, as well as strategies to meet new goals in the years to come.

Ok, the brain. I have been fascinated with the brain as long as I can remember. I read books on the brain and music, the brain and math, the brain and habit loops, the brain and [insert noun], even as a kid. I am not sure why other than I remember finding dreams very interesting, especially since I had intense nightmares and often knew I was dreaming but could not wake up. You know, normal kid stuff. Or so I thought. But I will try to contain myself from nerding out on you about all things brain, or we will all be in our 50s and beyond before you can read this. Instead, I will keep things relatively simplified and concise when it comes to picking out a few areas to discuss in how the brain can assist us in good routines, habit change, and goal achievement.

Oh! Before we dive into the parts of the brain I allude to, I want to share with you my first actual glimpse 'into' the brain. It was the first day of gross anatomy in physical therapy school. It's what you would picture. One expired body on each table, soaked in formaldehyde, and patiently waiting for us to meet them. There were 4 of us to each table to start. It turned out that the table to which I was assigned supported a body that was face down and we were supposed to start with them face up. So, the 4 of us were instructed to simply flip the body over. Sure. As you do. So, we did this in one relatively quick motion as instructed. I happened to be on the upper half closest to the head. As the head met the table, face up, the top half of the skull popped off, barely missing my own head, and it hit the floor spinning like a top. They had forgotten to mention that it had been removed and replaced to cover the brain until we got to that part of the body in class. In my startled and somewhat nauseated state in the moment that the skull flew off, I thought that the whole head had popped off. Keep in mind, this was our first moments of the first day of what was the first time most of us had ever seen (or smelled) a cadaver.

Needless to say, I rescued the skull and returned it to the

owner. Just as I was fitting it back on, I caught my first real glimpse of the brain. It was hard to believe what I was seeing could actually do all the things our amazing brains can do! That was a startling introduction to it, but I will certainly never forget it. Our glimpse into the brain in this book will hopefully be less flying skull and nausea and more 'oh interesting!' while sitting in your favorite chair and sipping your favorite beverage. Or, that's how I like to picture y'all. Yes, I still like the word y'all, even though I rarely get to hear it in California. But when I do, it makes me go awww.

Ok, let's dive in. The brain has 2 halves, left and right. I like to start with the basics, but then very quickly get to specifics. So, here we go. The more 'primitive' part of the brain is deeper and closer to the brainstem. Some refer to it as our reptilian brain, but basically think of the primitive (evolutionarily) part of your brain as your more survival-style part of the brain (fight or flight, etc). So, cheers to our primitive brain getting us to this point! The more outer layers of the brain involve more of the complex thinking (decision making, creating new things, etc).

The primitive part of the brain also controls our automatic behaviors, such as breathing. These are things that we generally do not have to think about on any conscious level. Thankfully. In terms of fight or flight responses, this would be the part of the brain that reacts, say, to an unexpected loud noise near you, which causes you to startle. It sets off a physiological reaction as well (increased heart rate, blood flow to your muscles in case you need to run from danger, etc). These are all incredibly helpful if you really are in danger of course, but it happens even when you are not because the primitive brain does not know the difference.

So, the primitive brain is key for survival responses and automatic behavior responses. Here is where it gets interesting for us. This part of the brain also includes our ability to store learned patterns (habits) and access them without thinking about it.

An even more specific part of the primitive brain that applies to automation is the Basal Ganglia. It is now understood that the basal ganglia plays a big role in automation that is more like autopilot, as opposed to fight or flight automatic behaviors. The basal ganglia is key in storing and recalling learned behavior patterns, much like what we sometimes refer to as running on autopilot. These behaviors include things like tying your shoes, putting on a seatbelt, the process of walking, even aspects of operating your car. Once you learn the pattern to create the movements to make whatever the activity is happen, you don't have to think about the details of how to do it anymore. Your brain and body just carry it out for you as a pattern.

This can be something pretty complicated when you think about all the things that have to coordinate in your body to walk. Imagine having to think about how much bend your knee needs to clear your toe from scraping the ground every step so you don't trip. And that's just a tiny piece of all that has to happen between your hips, knees, feet, let alone your abdomen and upper body for counter movement and stability. Otherwise you would fall over just from one part of your body moving forward without the rest reacting to keep your balance. I could go on and on. But, you get the point. Unless you have an injury that forces you to change your pattern or re-learn it, most of us don't have to think about all these things every time we walk across the room. So, hooray for the basal ganglia!

At some point in life you had to think about and learn these things in order to successfully walk without assistance. With repetition they became stored patterns to some extent, and your basal ganglia could help take over. I actually remember the first time I walked. I know people say you can't generally remember things before something like age 2 or 3, but all I can say is I do. I remember walking across the grass in the front yard of our house, thinking left right, left right, don't fall, left right all the way to my dad's outstretched hands in front of me. And the weirdest part, I remember it so clearly. I don't know how or why that is possible, but then, there are so many more things in my life I can't explain so... I just throw that one in for kicks! I asked my dad about it at some point. He was skeptical of course, but also said my description of where it happened and how I described it was accurate. The brain is a mysterious thing. We can leave it at that!

Our stored automatic behaviors are extremely important for us to function in our everyday lives because it frees us up to think about other things we are doing that take decision making and complex, conscious thought to achieve. We will revisit this concept later when we get more into habit change, building routines, and achieving things like fitness, health, and life goals. I just wanted to give you a little insight, or reminder, into how the brain handles all this at once.

Now let's talk about the brain when it comes to information overload! We know that automation helps 'free up' some brain space for other processing. And, there is SO MUCH input coming in every second. In order to not short-circuit ourselves, we have to have ways to filter the constant stream of information entering our brains. Otherwise, we would be completely useless amidst the chaos of overstimulation. There is a part of the brain called the reticular activating system (RAS) that helps with this, but for now I want to zero in on the concept of what I call 'noise' and how we can cut through that to actually 'think.'

In order to really even consider what we want out of life, where we currently are on that spectrum, and if/how we want to change or improve something specific such as our fitness or well-being, we have to first give our brains a genuine 'break' from the noise around us. This noise is both literal (people talking to us, phones making text sounds, cars honking on a busy street, etc.), visual (phones lighting up to show a text even if it is on silent, TV on in the background, etc.), and internal (wandering thoughts about your to-do list for the day, feeling like you should be doing other things, work or family stress, etc.). These are all things that our brains are constantly trying to process. We can get stuck in our daily 'grind' or routines (both mentally and physically) that are not necessarily serving us in the most helpful way. Unless you stop and take a look at these things and really consider how they are serving you in your life, you may waste a lot of energy and time unknowingly (or knowingly) hindering yourself from getting what you really want out of life.

So, my advice is: Just Stop.

I mean this on two levels. One, consider this, your time in your 40s, as a time to really stop and evaluate your life and goals so you can be sure to give yourself the best foundation for moving positively forward. Two, take some time to literally stop and eliminate the noise around you so you can truly, effectively evaluate these things. Easier said than done, I know. But, essential for real, lasting change that you actually want on a deep level.

Once you take some time to dive into your brain, you can take inventory of what's going on in there. Your 40s are a perfect time to do this in full. You have lived enough and experienced enough and gotten to really know yourself in ways that your 20s and 30s didn't quite cover. You have maybe had tragedies (and comedies) that you can reflect on that help put things in perspective when it comes to the bigger picture. By the time you reach your 40s, most of us have a strong sense of who we really are, what we really want, and what is no longer serving us towards that, even if it did at some point in our lives.

You also may be experiencing new or more body-breakdown issues that remind you of your mortality a bit more often! All of these things, combined with health problems, hormonal changes, and general life fatigue can send some of us into a state of WTF, seemingly all at once! All the more reason to see this as an opportunity to take control of what you CAN take control of in your life and set yourself up for your best shot at living every day you have left to its fullest. Or at the very least, get yourself back on the trajectory that helps you do this.

Whatever has been your journey so far has led you to now. And it all should be celebrated (even the tough stuff, because well, you are still alive and most likely stronger in some way because of it). It all adds up to where you are right now. So, let's take a good hard, honest look at what now looks like. Only you can take true inventory because this includes a lot of how you perceive yourself and how you think about yourself and your life so far. Be objective as much as you can, not judgmental of yourself. This is not to berate yourself for all the 'failures' or missed opportunities, or anything of that sort. This is actually just a time for information gathering on yourself. Sounds intrusive. But, hey, it's you observing your own brain. No one else has to get in there. In fact, best if you keep others' opinions out of this completely when you do this.

Here's the deal. Just stop, look in, and listen. Pay attention to your thought patterns. Tune in to what things run on repeat in your brain. Are they positive? Negative? What do you tend to dwell on? What do you tend to (try to) ignore? Relationship status? Job happiness? Family issues? Do you have 'nagging' thoughts? Things you want to change about yourself or your situation? Things you want to do before you die? Things you just want more of in your everyday life?

Pay attention to all these 'inner voice' conversations you're having with yourself. If there are repeated ones, or ones that you tune into specifically, write them all down. Yes, actually write them down. Like, on paper. Get it out of your head and onto paper. Don't think too hard, just write whatever comes to mind or whatever gets repeated, or whatever your gut tells you to write. Once you're done, go through and put a 'P' if it's a positive thought and 'N' if it's a negative thought. Add them up. It will give you an idea of what's going on in there on a daily basis. If they are ALL 'N's... well, don't feel terrible about yourself (duh, that's one more), just think 'well, I'm consistent!' This is all about information gathering, not criticism of your own overworked and still functioning-like-crazy brain.

Next 2 lists... make a more concise positive and negative list, drawing from your original script. List 5 positive things that you know your inner-self truly believes about yourself or your circumstances. This could be things you like about your personality, your body, your life, etc. Positive things you know and believe about yourself:

1.

2.

3.

4.

5.

If you didn't have 5 positives on the first go, then mine for them now. Now list 5 negative things you know your inner-self truly repeats (thereby 'believes') about yourself. These may be things you tell yourself you are not good at, things you feel you keep failing at, things you tell yourself you can't do or achieve, etc.

Negative things you think and repeat about yourself:

1.

2.

3.

4.

5.

I know, this can be annoying to have to stop (yep) and actually write and think intentionally about things you may not feel like thinking about… but, if you want life change, you first need mind change. It is just the way it is. I know, I had to experience it to believe it thoroughly myself! Ok, cheers to completing your 3 lists of brain inventory! If I was with you in person, I would hug you or cheers you (your call) for actually getting it done.

Doing this will give you a sense of your running thought streams going on that you may not even realize are highly affecting your ability to be who you want to be or do what you want to do. It is important to take a look at this before you try to change or add anything new or important into your life habits. It is crazy how much your subconscious thoughts actually determine your results.

Getting a thorough understanding of the current 'situation' in your brain is a lot like what I would do when I was treating patients in physical therapy. Before I could go about helping or solving the 'problem,' I would gather all the information available to me first, so I could figure out the best, most efficient way to help the person. This included knowing the current underlying feeling regarding the pain or injury, how it affected their thoughts about themselves or what they could do in the future, and a good idea of what may be the 'mental' obstacles in achieving their goals/ getting back to what they wanted to do.

The ability to be consistent and 'compliant' with any home exercise program or routine involved devising a way to make it easier on each person depending on their individual situation both physically and mentally. It matters with outcomes. Any thorough physical therapist would agree with this I am sure! Attention to details like these was key for effective and efficient recovery, not to mention lasting results!

It all starts with a thorough self-evaluation in order to set yourself up for success, meeting your goals, and solving problems/overcoming obstacles along the way. So, think of all of this as your initial (brain) evaluation. We will get to the physical (body) evaluation in Part II of this book. For now, get to know, or reconnect with, the True You. I say 'true you' because this is all about YOU, what you think, and how you feel. It is not about what others think or what others think you should feel or what others want, frankly. This is 100% about you. This is about being honest with yourself and starting to tune in to your inner voice, as well as your (current) thought patterns.

This leads us to your next list. I hope you like lists! This one is short. Write down the 3 things you used to like to do most as a kid. For ease, you can center it around age 10, give or take. List 3 things that you remember truly enjoying when you were a kid. If you could spend your time doing what you wanted as a kid around age 10, what would be your top 3? Top 3 things I liked to do as a kid:

1.

2.

3.

Now, write down your top 3 things TODAY.

Top 3 things I like to do today:

1.

2.

3.

I know, this can be hard. Don't worry about leaving something out, just, if you had to choose your top 3 for now, what would they be? If you had time to do what you truly enjoy doing right now, on a regular basis, at 40-something you, how would you spend your time? And just for added clarification, these are things that True You would choose to do. I am not talking about what sounds good or what others think you should do, but what you deep down enjoy the most regardless of any other circumstances around you.

Meaning, 3 things that don't rely on or involve any other person in your life. I know, that sounds harsh. But, these are things that don't involve your family, your spouse or partner, or any particular person currently in your life. It could involve other people in general, but not a specific person. These are things that would apply and make you happy out of pure enjoyment personally, no matter what/ who is in your life. This gets you closer to True You. Relationships change, people come and go in your life, and life circumstances change. These are just 3 of your current happiness-activities. They can change, there can be way more than 3 realistically, but pick 3 for now.

Doing this helps you reconnect with yourself and what you really enjoy doing. It taps into what makes you feel calm or excited or well, happy. It is your list, there is no right or wrong. I would think about it as 3 things that if you could do them every day for the rest of your life, that idea would make you feel extra happy or relieved or whatever word suits you. Put simply, these are things you love to do, no matter who is in your life. For me, I would say: 1) going to the beach 2) playing the drums 3) hiking/walk in nature.

Now that you have taken some time to peer into your own brain and reconnect with True You, I want to let you know something quite celebratory. You can be your own brain boss. We will get into this more in Chapter 2, but it is liberating to start taking charge of your own thoughts. I know that sounds weird, but it is true. Just like you can control your own actions/reactions, you can learn to take charge of how you see yourself, what you tell yourself in your subconscious, how you see your life, and how you choose to move forward in this journey.

How you think determines how you act, so if you truly want to change something in your life, this is great news! You just have to learn new thought habits (just like learning new body habits) and direct your brain to seek out ways for new action. I am sure you have probably seen or heard this before, but it is one of my favorite Albert Einstein quotes: 'The definition of insanity is doing the same thing over and over again and expecting different results.'

Your thoughts are more powerful than you might realize. I am sure some of you DO realize this and have experienced it yourself. But, I am not just talking about this in the 'law of attraction' and the 'good vibes to the universe' kind of way, although I love both of these as well! I am also talking about the you-can-train-your-brain-to-work-for-you kind of way. This is referring to the part of the brain mentioned earlier that helps filter information for you (the reticular activating system). Since your brain can only process so much information at a time, the RAS helps filter all the input.

If you train your thought patterns to align with things you actually want/desire, then your brain will take notice of things that apply to what you want, so you can be more aware of opportunities that can actually help you or assist you or remind you of these things. This is a huge advantage when you're trying to make a change or go after something.

But here is the important part: your brain does not know the difference between the something you want and the something you DON'T want. So, it will help you most to think of things and create thought patterns around the things you want, not the things you don't want. Otherwise, without you knowing it, your brain may be sending things your way (and to your awareness) that assist you in doing exactly what you don't want. The take-home here is when you are training thought patterns, make sure you are training yourself to think about what you DO want, not what you DON'T want in your life.

This will all come together in helping you become the boss of your own brain. We will get into tools to help you transform old thought patterns, purge thoughts that drive you away from what you want, and assist you in ways you don't even have to think about! Good stuff!

CHAPTER 2

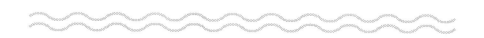

Re-Set

Now we want to look into how to actually re-set your old thought patterns and 'beliefs' about yourself and what you can accomplish. To change a thought you must first identify it. That's where all the thought downloading and brain inventory from Chapter 1 comes in. See what's there first and identify it. Next, you want to investigate it a bit. Ask yourself if this thought is actually serving your best interest. Maybe it served you in some way at some point in your life, but you are interested in you now. So, ask if it is serving you in terms of what you want out of life, or what goals you want to achieve. If it is not, then you need to challenge it. Is it true? Is it an actual fact, or just something you tell yourself based on your previous experience or based on self-doubt? Dive into why you think you 'hear' this thought pattern.

This is part of challenging it. You need to think about why it is there in the first place. Did other people tell you you couldn't do X? Did your parents tell you you couldn't do X? Did you try to do X and fail? You can ask the best questions because chances are you know the answer already, if you dive into it and if you give yourself a chance to be honest with yourself. It's worth the work of investigating this so that when a negative thought tries to creep back in later, you can remind yourself it is not a fact, just a repeated pattern.

Once you have identified the thought, challenged its truth, and realize it is just something attached to your past, now you can replace it with a current and actually beneficial thought. This part is good to work on, because just like with body habits, it is easier to replace an old habit with a new one as opposed to just trying to eliminate it completely. It tends to want to hang around if it is not well-replaced. So, you can just modify the old thought with your new one. We will get into this more in depth but realize it can be done and can be quite effective if done with intention. And this is the key: **you are creating a new thought to get repeated and 'learned' by your subconscious, so you want to make sure it is exactly what you want.** Otherwise, you are letting your brain be the boss of you. It will just continue to run on old information or negative past experiences and in no way assist you. In fact, it will continue to hinder you.

Thought habits are like body habits in another way. To make them stick, you have to make the effort to 'learn and repeat' the new habit persistently and consistently enough… reps reps reps… until it can be 'stored' and become your new 'automatic' subconscious thought habit. To do this, yep, reps. I know, rep-ing your brain sounds exhausting, but it works. And it is not like you have to do it all day long. Please don't. That WOULD be exhausting! You can think of it like any other exercise. You want to strengthen your thought muscles, so, start small and don't over-train. The easiest thing to do is just write down, say, 3 new thought patterns. Have it somewhere you will see it twice per day. Repeat it out loud or in your head 5-10 times. But, be INTENTIONAL. Don't do other things, concentrate on it for that moment and repeat. Do this every day. I'm sure that sounds weird to some of you, but it is easy to do and quick. Just be consistent and repetitive. An easy way to 'create the habit of creating this habit' is to have it on an index card by your toothbrush. If you brush twice a day, this will be an easy reminder. Plus, you have to be standing there staring at yourself anyway, so effective AND efficient. My favorite! But, do it however you like. Just do.

This is all very easy in one sense, but just like most new habits, it is harder than it sounds to make it become routine. So, just remember that this is all worth doing because you are now in charge and are reprogramming what will serve you tremendously in the future.

This leads into why this is so important when it comes to getting results, whatever they are for you. What you think determines how you feel about the area in your life that you are addressing. Whether it is your fitness level, your nutrition, your job goals, or your bucket list items. What you think about yourself and your ability to achieve it or whether you feel you deserve to achieve it, or whatever might be running in the background for you, determines how you feel about it.

What you THINK determines how you feel. What you FEEL about it, determines your ACTIONS towards that goal. And what actions you take determine your RESULTS. I was introduced to this model of thinking: Circumstances -> Thoughts -> Feelings -> Actions -> Results by a stellar business and wellness coach, TaVona Boggs, when I hit some road blocks while starting my own business. The C-T-F-A-R Model was developed by Brooke Castillo, the CEO and co-founder of The Life Coach School. It is a simple concept to understand, but when actually used on yourself in earnest, it can be quite eye-opening and effective. The trick is changing the THOUGHT to create the results you actually want. It starts there.

For instance, let's say you want to lose 10 lbs. Let's say you have tried, but failed. Or, you have succeeded, but then you were unable to maintain it. This maybe has happened multiple times. You might be subconsciously thinking 'I can't lose 10 lbs.' even if you consciously say to yourself 'yes, I want to lose 10 lbs!' So, your running thoughts in the background will be saying you can't, and this will make you feel disappointed or doubtful or whatever feeling you might have around losing weight. So, this translates into actions that don't fully support you doing this. This could be complete inaction as well. So, your actions may be attempts at reaching the goal (or no attempts), but they may not be realistic or sustainable or well-planned enough to reach your goal in the grand scheme. So… the results are exactly what your subconscious is saying is true. You can't lose 10 lbs and/or maintain it. And, those thoughts just keep recycling and working against you ever getting there.

Think about this. Self-doubt is a habit. If you constantly tell yourself you can't do something, it will get planted in your subconscious as 'fact.' It will work against you. Your brain will pick up on all the things that happen (or might happen) that support this 'fact.' And because it is your running thought, it directs your feelings about whatever that something is towards defeat, inadequacy, or disappointment. These feelings direct your actions regarding that to something either towards inaction or inadequate action. This means your action, or lack thereof, leads you to the results that support your original thought of 'I can't do X.' Then your brain stores this as more 'proof' that you are right. Here's the kicker. We all want to be right… so, your brain gets to congratulate you on once again being right that you can't do X. And the loop continues.

You wouldn't think of failure to achieve X as a reward (because your conscious thought is that you want the opposite), but to your brain and the nature of thought habits, you are rewarding your need-to-be-right part of the brain. You are continuing to prove it 'right' by getting the same (unfortunate) result. If you got a different result, the brain would see it as cognitive dissonance. The brain does not like cognitive dissonance, so it wants the results to line up with the subconscious thought.

Let's recap some things so far. To 'purge' old thought habits, you instead want to replace the old ones with new INTENTIONAL thoughts. Just like with body habits, at first it takes conscious decision-making to do this. You decide on the new thought that will serve you better. You repeat the new one until it is 'learned' by the subconscious. Your subconscious will eventually code this as your new 'reality' and repeat it automatically for you. Your brain starts acting in your favor by using the new thoughts, or beliefs, to direct your actions as well as picking up on things around you/ opportunities that help you get there. Now, all things up there are working FOR you, not AGAINST you! It's like magic! Or can be, if you really make the brain-change a priority. You will drive yourself insane, or at least to major frustration (and thereby inaction or inadequate action) by keeping the same old habits. See Einstein quote on insanity again! If you instead transform your thoughts to match the results you truly WANT, then you are setting yourself up to actually succeed.

This is obviously just a piece of getting the results you want, but if you skip this step, you are setting yourself up to fail. Right from the start. Ouch. So, you may truly, deeply want something, work crazy-hard to get it but all along the way your subconscious does not match your conscious desire. So, no matter how much you desire it and how much action you might take, it's a faulty plan in that you are not giving yourself a fair shot at getting there. Help you to Help you. Honestly, it is pretty amazing what you can do for yourself that no amount of time reading about it or joining different gym classes or trying different diets can achieve. When it comes to efficient, effective, and lasting results, the brain is the master at it. Get clear on what you want, know why you want it, and make the active decision to align your thoughts with it. PS if you feel like I keep repeating myself a bit... um, yes, I am! It is not an oversight or a case of writer's circle. It is repetition at work!

Now let's look back on what you listed as your 3 favorite things to do as a kid. Pick out one that still rings true. If none of them apply in any way to what you like to do today, modify it to something you still enjoy. This would be something you used to like to do and you would still enjoy, but you 'grew up' and concentrated on adulting so much that it got lost along the way. Or shelved. Or back-burnered. Or completely buried under all things 'have to do.' Let's say you liked to play basketball. Do you still play at all? Are your knees absolutely enraged if you even think about running up and down a hard court? Well, here's the thing. Modification. Whether your body wants to play full-on basketball at a competitive level is not the question. Did you like to shoot the ball? Maybe you would re-enjoy exactly that.

If you find yourself coming up with excuses right off the bat, that's fine. Listen to them. Your thoughts might be 'I don't have time' or 'I don't have a court near me' or 'my knees hate running, so

I can't play.' Ok. Let's break this down. If you physically cannot bend your knees at all, yes, that would be a 'fact' at the moment that would make this harder than most. Although, even bigger physical barriers can be addressed if you really want to do something. I am sure you have seen the amazing people playing basketball in wheelchairs. Awesome! But let's say you just know running on a hard court is not a good option for your knees (I mean, I would agree), that's fine. Chances are, if you really liked basketball, you probably really enjoyed the shooting part just as much as running around and dribbling. So, if you replace the 'I can't play ball because my knees hate running' with 'I enjoy shooting hoops and my knees are fine with that,' you can purge that excuse very quickly. Next excuse please... 'I don't have time.' Ok, replace 'I don't have time' with 'I can take 30 minutes a week to shoot hoops because I love it!' Boom. Excuse #2 purged. And, that's just a minimum if you want, obviously. It is just to illustrate that if you want something back in your life and you are extremely busy, there are still ways to integrate it back in. And you should. If it gives you an extra shot of JOY in your life, then it's totally worth working it back in. Start small. Small things can make a huge difference in happiness level overall. Also, if you try to stuff too much in your schedule at once, you will just feel stressed that you 'need to do other things' and not enjoy it. Just reintroduce it in a pleasant, joy-moment kind of way to start, if time is a big issue right now.

Next excuse. 'I don't have a court near me.' Two things here: 1) once you start thinking that you WILL play and CAN play, often your brain helps you out on the filtering side of things. You may notice the next day on your way home from work a perfect little outdoor court. Or you may see one literally 2 blocks away from your house that you never noticed. You may have passed either one a bazillion times, but never noticed it. Yep…brain now activated and working for you!

It's funny how this works. Sometimes the most obvious things are never noticed, let alone small things like that. I used to commute 40 miles to and from work every day on a major interstate in the middle of Missouri. One thing about the middle of MO… not a lot going on along that route except a lot of cows and an occasional exit sign. After years of this commute solo, I jumped in with a co-worker friend to carpool. When we got to work, she mentioned something that 'we had seen' on a billboard on our way to work. I said, 'what billboard?' She said 'uhhh, the HUGE BRIGHT YELLOW billboard, which is basically the only thing you see every day on that drive!'

Once she pointed it out, it truly was shocking I had never seen it. Of course, I saw it in all its massive yellow glory pretty much every day after that. But see, it didn't have anything to do with my life or trigger anything to do with me, so it got filtered out with all the other things I didn't 'see' on any given day. I love cows, probably because my mom loved them, and they would remind me of her and how they would always make her smile. So, most likely I saw every cow in a 40-mile drive, but not a big yellow billboard. Now, if that billboard had the upcoming tour schedule for U2, I would have noticed it immediately and every day afterwards (even with all the cows around)! My brain would have activated to alert me to something I wanted to know so I could start planning ahead for the next Dublin show. Just sayin', our brains know what drives us, or what we want it to look for. That billboard could have been pasture-green and asphalt-grey, and I would have definitely still seen it/registered it!

Reminder: Think in terms of what you DO want, not what you DON'T want.

Your subconscious brain doesn't know the difference.

I bring this up here to give you a few examples. If you are feeling anxious or stressed out, don't think over and over 'I want less stress in my life.' Instead think 'I want more calm in my life' or 'I want more relaxation time in my life.' This applies to all goals/ habits, including thought habits. We can apply this even more specifically to an earlier example about losing 10 lbs. Even though you know you want to lose 10 lbs. and that is your goal, try to put your repeated thought habits in the positive. You could say 'I want to weigh X number of lbs.' or you could say 'I want to be more fit' or 'I want a more toned waistline' or any number of things. Just remember it's even better if you can put your thoughts towards the positive and stay away from the 'negative' or 'less of' when you are 'training' your brain. Think 'more Abs!' instead of 'less Fat!' because your subconscious brain with hear 'Fat!' I know it sounds crazy, but it's true. Of course, you know that increased fitness or better abdominal definition = less fat, but your subconscious does not.

Speaking of repetition, remember your thoughts grow stronger with reps, just like your body. So rep it. Write it. Say it. 'Play it' in your head. Do all 3. Rep it until it is your new baseline thought. Purge the old. There will be no place for it. It has been replaced. But it needs maintenance. Check-ins. Re-visit and take inventory, so you know what's going on in there. If an old one has snuck back in, rep it out. Keep at it. It takes intention and persistence, just like building muscle. You are building new thought muscle. Let the old one atrophy and concentrate on strengthening the new one until it naturally takes over. This happens in the body, too. The stronger muscles naturally take over certain actions.

While we are on the topic of repetition, intention, and persistence, I want to mention a few things about habit formation and the question of how long it takes to 'form' a new habit. There is no absolute answer to this because of so many variables and a lack of conclusive scientific evidence so far, but I will give my thoughts and personal experience, along with a few nuggets of information that are out there. There is a generalized belief/suggestion that it takes about 3 weeks. This actually came out of some observations by a plastic surgeon in the 1950's (published in 1960), who observed that it took a minimum of 3 weeks for his patients to adjust to certain changes body-wise. Although this has been deemed 'the 21-day myth' by many in the habit-formation world, I can say that in my experience 3-4 weeks does tend to jive with about how long it takes for a habit to start to 'stick'. I think of it as 2 stages: the start to 'stick' phase and the start to 'stay' phase. Yes, I know. Quite science-y.

A study done in 2009 suggested that on average it takes 66 days for a behavior to become automatic. Again, there are so many variables to consider, but this may be a piece of why so many 60 to 90-day programs are successful. In my experience, especially with fitness programs, 3 months is when it feels like the routine/habit is more solidified and will 'stay'. The best way I can describe this is that after doing a fitness routine for 3 months, I feel like it is ingrained enough that taking 'breaks' is no big deal.

I am sure more information will come forth when it comes to the brain, the body, and habit formation. It is an exciting time for discoveries in the realm of the brain and neuroplasticity. I look forward to what new information springs forth in the years to come! For me personally, I operate with the 'stick' and 'stay' guidelines as benchmarks. It has worked for me. But in the end, it sticks when it sticks and it stays when it stays. So, just monitor yourself and stay mindful.

I have experimented with habits and habit change A LOT in my own life over the years. I find it fascinating (obviously!), but it is also quite helpful when it comes to personal fitness routines or healthy-living routines, not to mention hugely helpful when treating patients over the years trying to educate and assist with home exercise programs. New routines are not easy, even if they are 'simple' when broken down. Even more challenging is trying to develop new routines that are progressive and often modified. In these scenarios, there are baseline routines and then there are things added or modified every week. I found that establishing a baseline routine first, then gradually adding to it, with attention to detail, was the most successful.

I found that establishing a baseline routine first, then gradually adding to it, with attention to detail, was the most successful.

I have found this to be true in pretty much all of my personal experiences with habits or new routines as well.

I experimented for several years in order to find, what was

for me and is now, my baseline workout routine to achieve and maintain the fitness level I wanted. I put the time in to figure this out for myself because I wanted to see what worked best for my body overall no matter what else might be going on in my life. And let me say, it has been tested for sure! I have had significant injuries, health problems, and major life changes (good and bad) along the way. We all have these things, especially if we are in our 40s! There are going to be obstacles and unexpected tragedies, injuries, and the list goes on. These things are going to happen. To get through unforeseen or unexpected events or life changes (even if they are good things like an opportunity to travel the world) that present themselves and still maintain your health/physical fitness, it takes some determination. If you already have a foundation of good habits, a good workout routine, and some basic health habits in place, it can make a massive difference in how you move forward during these times. And for some, it can thwart a downward spiral of fitness/stamina/health that never quite recovers. It is hugely important, especially as we get older, to get a good foundation in place.

When things throw you off your intended path, you just have to find ways to get back on track as quickly as possible. If it is an injury, it is important to find ways to modify your routine to allow healing to that area, while still maintaining the rest of you that is functional. Because, let me tell you, you WILL need the parts of you that ARE functional and fit to help the rest of you recover as much as possible. This is why having a solid foundation in place is so important. Whatever comes your way, you can use that solid foundation to support you and avoid losing all ground you have to stand on in the process. We will get into this more thoroughly in Part II of this book, but I wanted to mention it here because your mental foundation is a huge part of your physical foundation. You will hit (or have already) times in your life that will deeply rely on a solid mental foundation of knowing how to battle the tough/negative thoughts that will try to take over. And if they do, you will know how to identify and transform them to positive/healing thoughts. Keep this mental muscle strong because it will be tested. As we enter mid-life, we tend to get more and more tests! Yippee! I want to help you be as fortified as possible pushing through them.

Ok! Here is where I want to throw some 'mental fortification' tools your way. There are many many tools you could use, but I am just listing a few that I have used in my life that have helped me. There are many variations on all of these things and there is no right or wrong way for using them, but I will give you a few thoughts on each.

1) **Meditation/Quiet Time**
2) **Dream-wake Journal**
3) **Visualization**
4) **Intentional thinking**

The first two are amazingly helpful, what I would call more passive, tools. Meditation or quiet time for your brain is just that… you are trying to clear your brain of clutter, of noise, of thoughts. Dream-wake journaling is taking note (this could be written or mentally noted) of what your brain was thinking about right when you wake up or when you are in the first few minutes of coming out of slumber. The next 2 are more active tools. I will explain a bit more about visualization, but it is what it sounds like. And the fourth is what we have been discussing with intentional thought change or repeated thoughts that you have intentionally decided on. So you already understand the basics for that one.

I used to think I 'could not meditate.' Yep. Poor form. It wasn't until this year actually, that I finally decided to change that. What I realized was that I just had not decided fully to do it, so I 'failed' at it and I didn't see results. Shocker. I decided it would help me clear my head before going to bed, since I have a strong tendency for brain-on-fire when I try to go to sleep. What I discovered was that previously I had tried either for too long right away (which for me was anything more than 5 minutes) or wanted instant brain-not-on-fire or it wasn't 'working.' Again, poor form!

I started with just a simple 'quiet time' moment before going to bed. I will give you the details in case this is all new to you. I am sure for many of you it is not. Here is what I did. I sat on a comfortable pillow on the floor, legs crossed, back straight. I closed my eyes and just concentrated on breathing in and out. Not forcefully, just natural breathing. Of course, my brain was on fire, but I let it burn a bit and just noticed what was going on. Once I got the gist of the thoughts, I just 'breathed' them out one by one as they popped up. If there were repeat players, I just acknowledged they were back and breathed them out again. After about a minute or two, I was able to get chunks of 'black.' I had short bits of time that I was able to not think of anything, just breathing and not thinking. For me, it was like seeing black in my head. Actually, if I am more specific, it felt like seeing blackness, or just infinite universe. But either way, it was free of brain-fire. Astounding for me, because in the past, I could never even get to chunks of that. The more I do it, the longer those moments tend to last.

The key for me was doing it every day, right before bed. I also use it sometimes in the morning and I know a lot of people use it first thing in the morning to get a good 'start' for the day. All of these things are good. Use it however suits you, and as often as works for you. If you have never tried it, just pick a quiet place and time and try it for 5 minutes. Ideally, you make it a habit every day. It can do wonders for brain 'clutter' and to help you re-set. If you are stressed and 'stuck' on a problem, try it to give your brain a break from the problem-solving. Often it helps get you to the answer soon afterwards or at least quicker than if you just force-solve when you're feeling stuck.

If you are really 'not into meditation,' I get it. Just think of it as quiet time for your brain. A brain nap of sorts, but while conscious. Man, I loved nap time… never slept, but I sure enjoyed the quiet! For some people, meditation or quiet time is crucial to control anxiety and stress. It is interesting how it helps in both powering-down mode (before bed) and re-boot mode (in the morning to start your day, or to interrupt repetitive thinking/anxiety). Use it for all these things as you see fit.

Meditation is the opposite of intentional thinking, so use each of them for their purpose. Your brain will thank you for both! The end result for both can be getting closer to an answer to a problem or making major life changes. They are both important pieces to these things.

Visualization is an interesting technique I have had some experience with as well. I have used it since I was a kid, even though I had no real idea that was what I was doing per se. I don't ever remember anyone telling me to try it or why I knew to use it, but I started young. I used it specifically for sports and music. Visualization is just picturing yourself doing whatever the thing is you want to do or to do well. For me as a kid, I used it to 'practice' sports or music when I either didn't have time that day or if I was just trying to get better.

I can remember lying in bed 'practicing' free throws and 'practicing' a piece on piano. Not at the same time! I was not THAT advanced. I would picture exactly where my feet would be behind the free-throw line, exactly how many times I would bounce the ball, then hand placement, then the shot to the basket. I would picture every detail of every shot. The funny thing to me was that I would also miss the shot sometimes. It was when I would lose concentration at all, the shot would miss. So, I would concentrate until I hit at least 30 (I know!) in a row. If I missed, I started over. Later, I did this same technique with 3-point shots.

With piano, if there was a tough part of a piece I was learning, I would visualize my fingers playing it correctly. Over and over. Until I got it. It honestly didn't strike me at the time that this was anything out of the ordinary. And maybe it is not. I don't know. I didn't talk about it. In fact, I didn't really 'think' about it at all. Until years later.

I was playing basketball on the junior high basketball team. During practice we would shoot around of course, but not over and over. One day, I wanted to see how many 3 pointers I could make in a row since I hadn't tried it in years. I waited until everyone left the gym after practice. I started shooting. And shooting. I hit 33 in a row. I missed on 34. And, they were perfect swishes. So weird! When I missed and started to leave, I was startled by the sound of my coach's voice exclaiming 'WHAT?! Well, why aren't you shooting 3 pointers in the GAMES?!!' Ha! I said, 'Ok, I will shoot more.' He shook his head laughing and said 'Well, Ok!'

This was obviously a type of visualization with regards to a specific activity, but you can use visualization in a more broad way, too. You can simply picture yourself doing or living whatever life or goal or change you want to accomplish. Picture the details, too. What you look like, what you are doing, how you FEEL having accomplished or achieved whatever it is, etc. I know it sounds goofy, but it can be a very mysterious and effective tool, in conjunction with all your other thoughts and actions.

The last one I will go into now is the dream-wake 'journal.' This is another one that might sound odd to you, but I have been amazed at what I have discovered/tapped into with it. As I mentioned, it's the idea of paying attention to what your thoughts are when you first wake. If you can remember your dreams at all, take note of them as well. If you can't remember specifics in your dreams, then just lie there quietly when you first awake and notice what's in your brain. I have solved some particularly bothersome 'problems' by just listening to those first few minutes. It gives you an insight into your subconscious and what I will just call your inner voice. Dreams can provide this insight as well. It is really just paying attention to what you already know, somewhere deeper in your brain, that gets clouded or drowned out by all the 'noise' of the day.

On a side note of sorts, another interesting 'technique' I have experimented with when it comes to dreams is what I will call 'intentional' dreaming. There are other names for it I am sure, but this is not lucid dreaming. This is simply posing a direct question to yourself before you go to sleep. It can be about something you are working on, something in a relationship, something you are trying to make a decision about, or whatever you are grappling with in your life. Pose the question and then let it 'go' in the sense that you don't want to be consciously ruminating on it when you are trying to fall asleep. I know ALL about that part! That is it. Just ask and then release it to your subconscious to play with all night. I have gotten 'answers' in my dreams, when I first woke up, or shortly after getting up. And every time it has happened, I have been shocked. I shouldn't be by now, but I can tell you it amazes me every single time.

And this brings me to just the simple reminder to pay attention to your intuition. Your inner voice knows a lot. Way more than we give it credit for. In fact, it can answer most of your hard-to-make decisions pretty quickly if you can find a way to tap into it. Usually, we know what to do, but we don't want to commit to it because it means we lose out on something or we are afraid it is the wrong decision. This can be torturous. I can relate. For me, the biggest decisions in my life have come down to truly listening to what my 'gut' is saying and eventually going with that and never looking back. Hard to do. But, of all the guides we have, I truly believe it is the most important 'tool' we can use. You just sometimes have to dig really deep to hear it. That, and push away all the 'logical' reasons we want the other choice long enough to connect to our own built-in compass. It is your life. Only you know what truly makes you happy or fulfilled. You have one life. Live it true to you.

Tips:

1. What you THINK determines your RESULTS
2. Purge/Replace old thought patterns with new, BENEFICIAL thought patterns
3. Rep your brain with new thought patterns daily
4. Think in terms of what you DO want, not what you DON'T want
5. Think 'stick' (3 weeks) and 'stay' (3 months)
6. Pay attention to your INTUITION!

CHAPTER 3

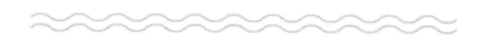

Mental Launch

Our mental habits are key to launching our physical habits. Our mental habits are also key to launching… well, our mental habits. Yep. Our brain habits will be integrated into accomplishing our body habits, and we will discuss this in more detail in Part II of the book. But, we now want to put into practice our mental habits, laid down as a foundation for what I will call mental fortitude! It will serve to help calm you, allow you to focus, give you mental energy, direct your thoughts (and thereby your actions) to align with what you truly want, and tap into your inner compass.

To make these seemingly simple 'routines' become a true habit, we need a plan. So, think about your daily schedule, whatever it is right now. I will keep this as doable and efficient as possible, and then you can build on it as you learn both the benefits and the way it works best in your busy (or not busy) life.

First, pick a time of day that suits you best for a quiet 5 minutes to yourself. For some of you, this is easy and some of you… I can only imagine how hard that might be. But, 5 minutes… find it! It is there, you just have to create it. The quiet part means no distracting noise, no distracting people, and no phones (unless you are using it for your 5-minute timer and in that case, silence other than the timer). I found that having a timer set, so you are not feeling the need to interrupt yourself just to see if 5 minutes is up yet, was most effective for me when I first started the 'habit.' Here's the great part - your job is to do NOTHING. Do the most 'nothing' you have ever done. Just sit up straight, on a pillow or the floor (or whatever you decide works better for you).

If you already meditate, then you are ahead of the game and don't need this part explained. However, it seems a lot of people have tried and 'failed' or try, but only occasionally when it can be 'fit in.' And then, there are many many people who have never tried (or wanted to, to be blunt). I fit into each of these categories as some point in my life. But, I just didn't 'get it' or realize I really needed it, or I tried and decided I 'couldn't.' And by 'couldn't,' I mean I had brain-on-fire and could not settle my brain even close to 'nothing.'

So, here are your instructions…Quiet your brain. Ha! I know, impossible! But do it anyway. Just breathe naturally, and as thoughts swirl, breathe them each away. And repeat. And repeat. And… see the last two sentences. By the way, I had very good English teachers and I know grammar and sentence structure… but, I prefer to write more closely to how I speak/think. Sorry, Ms. Fowler! You taught me well! Please don't take offense. I just needed to get that out there. Ok. Back to it. See… this is what it was like when I first tried to meditate… thoughts all over the place!

At first, it did feel impossible to me, to clear my head. But honestly, after just concentrating on 'seeing black,' or what looked like 'the universe' to me in my head, I was able to gradually get more clear (closer to nothing). It got surprisingly easier to do, even though I had a million things to do and think about. This is nap time for your brain. Remind yourself that you have the rest of the day (or next day, if you are doing it before bed) to let your brain be on fire. This is your official Time Out. Use it! Love it! Look forward to it. It is a much deserved and necessary break. And just like rebooting your computer when all tech-hell is going on, it gives you a chance to re-set.

Ok, so do this 5-minute meditation/quiet time/universe gazing/

brain napping… whatever makes you feel less awkward thinking of it as, so that you will do it Every. Single. Day. Ideally, you do this every day for 90 days before you let yourself balk. I know, days are busy and you're tired and people think you're weird and you can't think of 'nothing'… all the things. Now that we have gotten past the yawn-inducing list of excuses, just decide you will do it for your brain health. Reminder: you have ONE BRAIN. Let it rest for 5 minutes! It will thank you. And it will work even harder FOR you in the grand scheme.

Ok, excellent! You have made a realistic plan (5 minutes/day for 90 days), you have picked the date to start (today), you have made the decision to do it (all excuses crushed), and you are acting on it (Done). Cake! Not just a piece, the whole thing. Wait, don't EAT a cake, just sayin' … you've got this! Now I want cake. (Sorry.)

Congratulations! You have launched your first brain-happiness habit. I'm telling you, don't let the 'meditation is just for drum-circle Californians' thought deter you. Although my own example there cracks me up because… I am a drummer (set, not circle) and I do live in California… but even so, don't let any 'it's not for me' thoughts deter you. I wish I had made it a habit a LONG time ago. At the very least, try it for 90 days and then make the decision whether you want to keep it in your life-routine or not.

We talked about some other 'mental tools' besides meditation/ quiet time at the end of Chapter 2. As I alluded to earlier, I believe in 'baseline and build' to make new habits/routines sustainable and solid. So, I would suggest just getting 'quiet time' going and consistent in your day first before adding these others. But, if you're ok with more than 5 minutes added right away, then definitely feel free to do the next ones I discuss right from the start. They are actually all very 'short and sweet.' And this is the thing, they are not hard to do, it is just sometimes hard to make it a consistent and sustainable habit.

Ok, so the next one is visualization. Let's use a simple example from earlier, like you wanting to get basketball back in your life because you enjoy it and miss it. Visualization can work for you two-fold in this example. Take 1 minute each day to visualize shooting the ball (perfect swishes!) and visualize what you are wearing, the court (outside or inside, etc.), and the FEELING you have when you make each shot. Just that. 1 minute of picturing yourself doing the thing you want to do (your goal, pun intended) and how you feel doing it (happiness, movement feels good, coordination feels good, you feel good, etc). This will get your brain prepped in several ways to make this goal a reality. Your brain will 'look for' your perfect court near home, start reconnecting with the brain-to-muscle movements you stored long ago, AND your thoughts about doing it will drive your actions to get it back in your life. As I said, I like efficiency and effectiveness! 1 minute, 1x/day, every day.

I used a relatively 'easy' example of something you want to do/have in your life, but the same patterns apply to more 'complicated' goals or desires in your life. These 'mental tools' will serve you towards health/happiness daily habits, weekly habits, and bigger picture goals in your life (things like fitness level, your ideal job, your bucket list goals, or whatever else you truly desire in your life). BLAM! You have launched your second mental habit. It's quick, easy, and makes you feel good. That combo is hard to beat. If you are keeping track, we are up to 6 minutes of your day so far.

The visualization subject will change or morph over time, and as you reach individual goals, but the habit stays the same. 1 minute per day. Of course, you can do it more than once per day or longer if you are able. Or, do several rounds, with different goals. But, don't overwhelm yourself. Just pick one and get started. Another option is to use that minute for a 'bigger-picture' visualization. This is a broader version of visualization. You can picture yourself exactly how you want your life to 'look.' You would visualize your ideal place to live, your ideal job, what you look like/your health, and how you feel living this perfect-for-you life. Don't forget the 'feel' part. I know, it sounds weird, but keep it in the routine. Be specific in the details. The more details the better. Also, remember, this is YOUR dreamscape. This is not what you think you SHOULD want or what others think you should want, or what others in your life want. Nope! Every piece of it is what True-You wants.

Ok, on to the next brain habit. Again, you can add the next one after you have established the first 1 or 2, or you can start tomorrow! I say tomorrow because this is the dream-wake habit. I love this one! Think of it as what you do for the first 2 minutes of waking up. By the way, I don't love the waking up part, I just love the results it can produce! But I mean, you're groggy in the first 2 minutes anyway, so you might as well use this 'groggy' moment to your advantage. In fact, I would argue you are groggy in that moment for a reason - this one. This groggy state is when you can tap into your subconscious/intuition/inner voice/magical-ness. Uh huh. I'm not gonna lie, it has been magical at times.

Here is your easy daily habit spelled out. When you are first starting to realize you are waking up, try to tap into what you were dreaming about. Just see what you find. If you can't quite grasp it, you can try rolling back into the position you think you were in while asleep (if you moved as you woke). I know, it all sounds a bit weird. But this can sometimes remind you of what you were last dreaming. If you remember the dream, just take mental (or written) note of what it was, whatever you remember. If you don't remember a dream, then just 'listen' to what your thoughts are when waking, for the first 1-2 minutes. Also take note of these. That's it. Don't try to 'think,' just notice what your thoughts are. I am going to leave it at that in terms of 'what' to do, because I think if you start doing it, you will see what I mean without me trying to explain it too much.

If you pay some attention before you jump up and start the day and have all your conscious thinking strongly take over, you may notice you get some answers to some questions you have been grappling with, or you may just feel more clear about a particular thing in your life. If you don't experience anything like that right away, don't stop trying it. It may just be harder for you to access when you first start, or you may only experience/realize something every once in a while. Play with it and see what you discover. At the very least, you might enjoy seeing what your subconscious was batting around in your dreams. Some people would say our dreams are our truest insight into ourselves, if we pay attention.

Ok, for those 'trackers' in the crowd, we are now using $5+1+2 = 8$ minutes of our day for brain habits. You might feel you don't even have time to brush your teeth, let alone add brain habits (please brush your teeth!), but the rewards are more than worth the time. Besides, you have to brush your teeth so you can repeat your 3 new thought patterns you created in Chapter 2! Am I annoying you yet with all these brain habits? I hope not! But see, this one goes with something you are already doing as a health habit (teeth brushing), so no added time! Bonus! If any of this feels like too much all at once, just remember the 'baseline and build' strategy. You can always find ways and time for what's important to you in your life and this is the beginning - the mental foundation to have in place to support you in going after what's really important. Brain health is definitely key to anything else you want out of life, so make it a priority now. As we continue our life's journey, these tools will help us get through the rough stuff, keep pushing us towards the good stuff, and give us extra momentum towards the great stuff!

Speaking of the great stuff, I want to hit on a few other 'tools' for moving towards and celebrating the 'great stuff' in our lives. I will list them here and then give a shout-out to each:

1) **Gratitude**
2) **Goals**
3) **Contingency plans**
4) **Decision making**

I could write a whole book on gratitude (as others have)! It is one of those things that, even if you feel it, celebrate it, are highly conscious of it… the more you remind yourself of it (ahem, what I am doing now) the happier your life. Full Stop. Hands Down. No Contest. And so many other two-word combos I could think of, but will stop. Remind yourself. Truly celebrate what you have. Be grateful. Every. Single. Day. I know it can get lost in a really bad day or during a tragedy in your life. But, these are even bigger reasons to go there. Every Day. I know it is said by many people and in many ways, but the simple act of taking a moment to truly celebrate, let's say 3 things, that you have or had happen or you learned from today, is one of the most important things to do for yourself every day. Even the 'bad' things. You can find ways to learn from 'bad' things, or you can remember that if X (bad) thing had not happened today, I might have been in a different place and something much much much worse could have happened. You never know. That 'bad' thing may have saved you from a much worse fate. I tend to think of things this way. And for me, especially in some pretty extra-challenging times in my life, gratitude has saved me and preserved my happiness in many ways.

Gratitude is something that all of us, no matter how bad things are, can be grateful for… gratitude itself. Sorry to blow your mind here, but the fact that we have a brain that ALLOWS the ability to feel gratitude… and a body that can also FEEL gratitude… and all you have to do is remember it's there… well, the idea of NOT using it is tragic. Use it. Feel it. It's there FOR you, your health, and your happiness. No matter what. Needless to say, I am a fan!

On to Goals! I am almost paralyzed in what I want to say here because… so much to say… but in this part I just want to touch on the What vs Why concept in relation to goals. You obviously need to know What you want, in order to move toward it. But, it is also just as important to know Why you want it. The 'why' part is what will motivate you, sustain you especially when it gets hard, and solidify it once you're close/achieve it. I have found it's extremely helpful to 1) identify the 'why' when you establish you want something and 2) remind yourself of the 'why' throughout the process. Figure out what you want, why you want it, and then make a REAL plan to go after it.

This brings me to #3 - Contingency planning. Just as important as a 'real' plan, which involves being REAListic in your expectations of yourself, is making contingency plans for all the reasons (cough… excuses) that you know will pop up along the way. You know you best, so calling yourself out ahead of time is the best plan! Whatever excuses you might try to pull on yourself, try to cover those bases before you even put the plan in motion. It's just poor planning to not have a plan for all the things that will try to throw you off your… plan. Uh huh. Plan for your plan-busters before they even have a chance to challenge you in your weak moments! If you know your strategy to correct for, work around, or just plain crush all your upcoming excuses… well, now, you have a thorough plan. See, the thing is, there are going to be things you CANNOT predict and will have to work through/around, so get all the pesky predictable buggers out of the equation before you even meet them in real-time. Yep. It works. It's often the reason a 'perfect' plan does or does not succeed. Excuses and challenges are inevitable, so build in the adaptations/modifications/workarounds. Oh! And rewards!!

I could write a whole book about REWARDS, too! Build in rewards. Not only do they make for joyful moments along the way, but your brain loves and responds to rewards bigtime! Rewards also keep you on track and motivated. But mainly, be good to yourself! Reward yourself as part of the plan. Goals and plans are not about being miserable and depriving yourself of joy in life! You deserve to build in happiness, rewards, and celebration throughout because, duh…

life is short (!) so find ways to enjoy the journey along with the 'work' to get what you want. Integrating the two - that's the BIGGER goal.

Before we end this part of the book dealing with the brain, thought habits, and mental gloriousness, I want to say a few things about decision-making. Making a REAL decision is based on believing you can achieve whatever it is, aligning it with your true desires/beliefs, and holding yourself accountable. Think of a decision as a promise to yourself. Treat yourself like you would your best friend. Unless you are a bad friend, if you say you are going to do something, you follow through. You don't want to let them down. Well, don't let yourself down by making a 'decision' that you are not fully 'in.' Letting yourself down plays on your psyche and is cumulative as well. You will see yourself as unreliable, whether you consciously think this or not! This then feeds into your actions, creating more scenarios of not following through. Now your brain is 'rewarded' with being 'right' that you are unreliable. Boo! Instead, put yourself in a position to succeed, not fail, the moment you make a decision.

I have mentioned that I have had some challenges with decision-making in my past (understatement!), but I find decision-making quite freeing and rewarding. It can be hard to do if you feel it's the life-altering kind (who to marry or not marry, where to live, what to do with your life… the list is long…)! But once you make a decision, truly DECIDE to do (or not do) something, a massive weight is lifted. And then later, you sometimes really wish you had been able to speed it up! But 2 things with this: 1) maybe you just didn't have a grasp on tapping into your intuition, so it was well worth the wait to get there and 2) the quicker you can access that inner voice and decide, you are now released to move in the direction that serves you best. You can then get back on… or find… or redirect yourself TOWARDS what is best for you and happiness.

I recently heard a podcast that talks about what Brooke Castillo (The Life Coach School) calls 'Decision Debt.' It brings this home brilliantly. Get out of Decision Debt! Address any lingering decisions you have accumulating and are weighing you down. You may not even realize they are weighing you down, but they are. The sooner you do this, the sooner you are free from that weight.

All these things apply to big and small decisions in life. I am not saying it's easy to make a big decision (not at all)! But I do know it's not only good for your lower-stress health, but also allows you to actively pursue/correct your trajectory that you know deep down is right for you. And if you make a decision, and down the road realize you now know what's right for you in that area, it becomes a new decision. It is just a matter of 'recalculating' and making the next decision to get you back on track. As long as you are using your inner compass to guide you, there are no wrong decisions. They all lead you to where you are today. And today is good because … let's recap: you are alive, you've made it to your 40s, and you have a functioning brain which allows you to make decisions, make plans, make goals, feel gratitude, train your thoughts to work for you, and ultimately go after what makes you happy. Cheers to ALL that!!

Tips:

1. **5-minute Brain Freeze every day**
2. **1-minute Visualization every day**
3. **2-minute dream-wake journal every day**

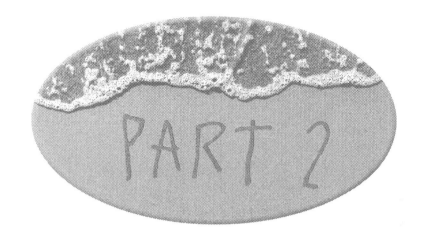

The Body: Gear Up

CHAPTER 4

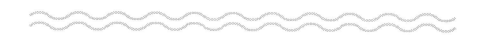

Body Baseline

Ok! Settle in. Find a comfortable chair. I have to say, this feels like a monster undertaking considering everything I want to say, everything I have learned, taught, discovered personally, and find truly amazing about the body. I will do my best to bring together all the concepts and body tips in a way that sparks new ideas and strategies for you to use as a foundation of healthy habits that will serve you for the rest of your life. Many are very simple in theory, and you may know many of these already but learning to incorporate them into your daily life is key. I hope to help you, remind you, and motivate you to find the key!

This chapter is about body baselines. In order to correct, create, and integrate good body habits into your life with lasting effects, we first have to take inventory (just like we did with your brain). We want to stop and 'look.' This is about paying attention to what your body is currently doing on a daily basis (and used to doing). This is not about berating yourself for being lazy or unfit or anything of the sort! We are information gathering.

First, let's look at your body 'input' habits. What you put in, or 'give' your body, is basically what it runs off of to… well, do stuff! This could be looked at in so many ways (and in more complex ways), but I have broken it down into 3 simple categories for our purposes:

1) **Food/Supplements**
2) **Hydration**
3) **Sleep**

I include sleep in body input because it is a big part of what you 'give' your body to run on. It helps your body recover and reboot each day, and it fuels you along with food and water. Of course, it does so many things when it comes to brain health, energy level, cell recovery, and the list goes on. Sleep is one of my favorite things! I haven't been able to get much of it until this year, and I know what huge toll it takes on the body (and mind) when it is a major challenge in one's life. I hope most of you have not been quite as drastically challenged as I have over the years, but I am sure many of you have felt the rough effects when you are deficient.

Food. What you eat, when you eat, and how much you eat are each worth taking a look at in your own routine, whatever that may be. Some people eat when they are hungry, some when others eat, some just because it's habit/time of day, and some very intentionally. All of these things play into whatever your current eating habits are. Due to health conditions, time conditions, financial conditions, etc., we may all do this differently. I just want you to take notice of YOUR eating habits so you know where you are starting (and can consider why as well).

Do you eat what you consider a healthy diet? Do you avoid certain foods that you know your body dislikes? Are you sugar-conscious? Do you have a stomach-of-steel and enjoy eating whatever you feel like? Do you eat at a certain time of day for meals? Do you take any supplements? Do you plan your meals or just go with whatever happens to be left in the frig? When you start paying attention to all of these things, you will start to get a better handle on your eating habits. Sometimes just taking note of these things will spur you to clean up your act a bit, without any significant work. For many people who are wanting to improve their intake habits, the simple habit of journaling itself sparks some pretty amazing changes. Charles Duhigg describes this brilliantly in his book 'The Power of Habit,' where he cites a 2009 study done by the National Institute of Health. 1600 people were asked to journal what they ate at least one day a week, nothing else, just journal it. After six months, those people that had decided to journal every day had lost twice as much weight as everyone else. By the way, if you haven't read 'The Power of Habit,' I highly recommend it! I loved it (shocking, I know)!

I am not suggesting you need to lose weight. But if you feel you do, keep food journaling in mind! I am not even saying what you should or shouldn't eat (I am not a dietician or nutritionist, so I leave that up to them when it comes to specifics), BUT I do know what habits have worked for me (or not worked for me) when it comes to eating schedules, what I choose to eat, and how much I eat. And, I continue to adjust and improve upon my own choices and 'intake' habits along the way. I have found the body starts letting you know more and more what it wants or absolutely does not want as I have entered my 40s!

I have discovered a few things personally that I think are worth mentioning here. Sometimes the most obvious things are skipped over in our daily lives. Ok, brace yourself. Eating healthier meals means you are running on better fuel! Yep. It is just that simple. Yet, so hard to do for so many. Second, taming the habit of over-eating is quite helpful. Again, so obvious yet so elusive! Oh, here we go. Eating slower, literally, helps digestion AND decrease the tendency to over-eat. And my more recent favorite, eating your last meal earlier in the evening gives your body a fasting habit that, for me, had great benefits all around. At first, I thought I would be hungry when I went to sleep, but that quickly was a non-issue. The hardest part was just making it happen. It takes some schedule-changing and some habit-forming persistence, but my body is WAY happier on all levels including sleep, digestion, and all the benefits that go with giving your body a 'fast.' Speaking of which, I always have a little moment of 'duh' when I remember where the word 'breakfast' comes from. These are all just simple suggestions to consider in your eating-habit life. In the end, do what works for you when it comes to diet. But remember, make your habits work FOR you, not against you. If you are trying to eat in a more healthy way, start looking at each of these things so you can get a sense of what your habits are (or that you even have them)!

When you start paying attention to your eating routines, you may discover some simple patterns. Do you have a 'snack' habit? If you know you tend to have a snack: 1) Are you actually hungry or just anxious or bored? 2) Is it a healthy snack or unhealthy snack? I mean, if you know you get hungry at around 4:00pm every day, but you are still at work and won't eat until 7:00pm, take notice. What are you choosing to eat? Are you even aware you are in this habit? What easy changes can you make to keep the same 'routine' if you want, but change the 'what'? I would also say take note of the 'why' because you could also change the 'what' to a short walk or some other activity if the 'why' is not actually hunger.

I want to go back to the habit of dinner 'time.' Just so you know, I do realize that there are challenges to eating earlier in the evening for all kinds of reasons that involve our varied schedules. I am not saying I always do this, but I took the initiative to 'make it a habit' for long enough to see 1) how I felt and 2) figure out ways to make it work in my schedule for the week. If you simply feel you do not have this option in your life, just eat as early as you can and avoid the later evening eating as much as you can. Of course, there are going to be days I choose to eat later, when there are special events, going out with friends, or whatever the situation. But here's the thing, I choose to give myself leeway for life-stuff and fun-stuff but, I operate overall on the new habit. And here is my personal strategy for not only eating habits, but also exercise habits… the 5/7ths rule.

I started using the 5/7ths rule for myself years ago when I decided I wanted to improve my fitness level. I will get more into this later, but it's just 5 days of 'healthy eating' and 'chosen exercise routine' and 2 days 'off.' Part of the reason I chose this schedule was that I am a realist with myself! I knew weekends tended to involve eating out, going out with friends, or trips. I also knew I didn't want to be so strict with myself that I left out things I truly enjoy. Nope! So, I started planning meals with more attention to 'healthier' foods during the work week, as well as working out 5 days during the week. Then I would do whatever variation I wanted on the weekend. BUT, key here is then being strict on making sure I kept to the 5-day part. It has worked for me and I still operate on these guidelines in my 'normal' routine. Now, in the bigger picture if I am on a trip or there is a particular event or anything that interferes, I just shift or adapt or alter it for those things. I don't force it when it truly does not make sense in the scenario, but I plan for those things ahead of time. And I celebrate them! I consider it a fun diversion and take full advantage of the special things in life in the moment. But, then as soon as I can, I get back to my 'routine.'

This is the thing. If you use, for example, the 5/7ths rule for your exercise routine OVERALL, then it is no big deal to take a few days off (or even a week or two if on vacation, etc.). It becomes a perfect balance of 'routine' for basic health, but full-on carpe diem when fun things come along! I will get into strategies that I use to keep the habit, or modify the habit, especially dealing with an exercise routine while traveling. The important thing is establishing your baseline. However you decide to do it.

The 5/7ths rule allows me to build in 'free' days and 'rewards.' This doesn't mean I eat terribly or sit and watch TV all day on my days off. Not at all, in fact, often I will hike or do some other fun thing on those days. And often, I still choose to eat a healthy meal on those days, it just gives freedom and variation along with the routine. Since then, I have also added the eating-earlier routine in a similar fashion. It really just comes down to percentage of the week I am doing certain things. It has worked wonderfully for me, even though it took some work to make it my 'normal.' Balance is what we are all looking for I think. Being kind to our bodies, but still kickin' it with fun and free times has worked for me!

I love scotch. I love wine. I love dark chocolate. I love Bolognese. I don't deprive myself of my favorite things. I just find ways to savor them more when I DO have them and reward myself with them! I am saying all of this to let you know I am not some perfect-eating, scoffs-at-anything-not-salad kind of person. Far from it! I just know what works for me in terms of combining a healthier lifestyle WHILE still enjoying what lights me up as rewardingly tasty! You will discover what works for you. Habits are the key. If you create a good baseline for yourself, you can then create the rewards that suit you. For some people, alcohol is a problem, and that would change the equation of course. We each have to figure out what a healthy balance looks like. And then, make it happen.

Supplements are something, much like meditation, that I didn't really 'believe' in until my 40s. I am not saying you should or shouldn't take any particular supplement. But there are ones out there that provide some pretty great benefits for many people. Again, I am not a nutritionist and don't pretend to be! I can just say that for me 1) omega 3s, certain 'superfoods,' and Vit C and D are working for me and 2) as we get into our 40s and beyond, I think it is worth considering whether your body may be lacking (and begging for!) some nutrients you may not be getting from your diet. Here is where I have to say, of course, consult your doctor or nutritionist on these things to find out what's right for you and any specific health conditions you may have.

On to HYDRATION! Ok, I will tell you that as simple as drinking water sounds it is one of my hardest-to-do basic health habits! This has always been 'a thing' for me. I don't get thirsty. It's weird. So, as long as I can remember I had to be reminded to 'DRINK WATER!' I mean, I could go all day long and not even think about drinking anything - not ok! I remember my mom would always ask me if I had had any water… not… had I done my homework (I think my parents knew I had that well-covered, for whatever reason), but had I had water. I also played sports (in the hot and humid south) and was very active, so this was even more important. And the challenge continued. I would occasionally even get an are-you-drinking-water phone call in college. And in grad school... or, after a big decision like say, getting... Dis-engaged after 8 years of... engagement...yep! Talk about Decision Debt! Ha! So, decision debt AND dehydration... hooray for me! But I digress. My point here is I had to create a 'habit' of drinking water. It seemed ridiculous, but I have to say, I have had to have many 'cues' along the way.

I worked in a physical therapy clinic in Puyallup, WA around 10 years ago. My friend (although we started this the day I met her, so my immediate friend!) and office manager would point at my water bottle that was sitting on my desk after every patient I treated. All day long, every patient. Thank you, Katie! You kept me hydrated for years!

So, my trigger for the habit was pretty awesome and consistent... Katie pointing at my water as soon as I entered her peripheral (even while she simultaneously answered phones/typed/scheduled patients). Once I left that clinic, I kept the same after-every-patient habit going. Sadly, I no longer had Katie's hilariously demanding pointer-arm (she is 6'3", so her arm seemed to span the length of the office to my desk), but the habit was already in place, so it worked.

This worked up until I no longer treated patients. So, I have since had to come up with more triggers/cues. Sometimes I use the alarm on my phone. I have even filled up a water bottle and put it 'in my way' so I would be sure to grab it if I was headed out the door. I know, ridiculous! But, as life routines change, sometimes you have to keep creating a new cue!

Hydration is extremely important for your health, so I make a major effort towards this habit. I also give this example because what is maybe easy or natural for many of you, happens to be a challenge for me. We are all different in what habits need more attention, or continued monitoring. So, just see where you stand on each of these and take note of what needs some love from you.

Ok, on to SLEEP! Wait, not you. Or, I mean, sure, if you prefer to continue this tomorrow. Oh man. I will not go into too much detail with my wrestle with sleep over the years, because: 1) you would think I am an alien and 2) you would wonder how in the world I have survived to even (not really) tell the story and 3) you would probably not trust anything coming out of what was an extremely sleep-deprived human brain for so many years!

I will just say this: sleep, people! Whatever you have to do to improve your sleep habits, if you have issues with this important re-fueling process, do it. Try the pre-sleep meditation I mentioned. Try improving your pre-bedtime routine. Take a look at your diet and timing of it. Consider whether your body is missing or depleted in any particular vitamins/minerals. Try all these combined. For me, all of these things combined have been a piece of what has been an incredibly-improved-after-trying-everything-in-the-past situation. I guess that's the other thing to remember. Even if you have tried or think you have tried some of these techniques in the past, your body may be ready to accept them now.

I will mention a few pre-bedtime habits that have assisted me in the process, besides the 5-minute power-down meditation. I am sure you know of or have already tried some of these. Be aware of the blue light thing. This is what comes off of your computers/phones/TVs, as well as a lot of lights in your home. Ideally, you 'disconnect' from your computers and phones several hours before bedtime. If you are not ready to do this, at the very least you can set your computer and phone to the 'night shift' setting. I happen to have an iPhone and a Mac and could easily change the settings on both. On the iPhone, it was under Settings—>Display Brightness—>Night Shift. I have mine set to 'sunrise to sunset' setting. As it explains, it automatically shifts to less blue-light display (and you can manually adjust to a 'warmer' setting within that mode). More 'warm' just means you are exposed to 'less blue and more red' light from the screen. We have receptors in our eyes that, when exposed to the blue light spectrum, signal hormonal and chemical responses in our bodies to 'wake up.' This is what happens with sunlight (the sun is our natural blue-light alarm clock) and then what happens in reverse when it gets dark. Tapping into our natural circadian rhythm by reducing blue-light sources after dark, we can help our bodies power-down!

You can try to use our natural light/wake cycle and natural dark/sleep cycle to your advantage in big ways when it comes to sleep habits. It is not the easiest thing to do logistically, but you can at least improve upon your current exposure at night. TV/computers can be a tough one for some people, if you like to relax with a Netflix or TV show before bed. You may feel you can power-down better with this routine, so in that case, try the night shift option (and at least keep some distance from the TV - the closer you are, the more exposure).

Oh! I haven't tried this yet, but why keep it from you… there are blue-light glasses that you can buy that block the wakey wakey blue light coming your way! I plan to look into that as well, since watching an old episode of Sex and the City is kind of my pre-bed jam. I might as well give in to ANOTHER pair of glasses (I finally gave in and got reading glasses) now that I am in my 40s. Nobody told me that you wake up one day at 42 and can no longer see out of your previously 20-20 eyeballs! I might as well look into fancy blue-light busters, too, if I am getting used to having a foreign object hanging out on my face already. I know, I am very grateful I was lucky enough to have close-to perfect vision until my 40s. I am sure many of you were not that lucky.

Ok, let's recap. Take body 'input' inventory on yourself. Take a gander at your diet habits, your hydration habits, and your sleep habits. Start thinking about which ones need a little tweaking. I will venture a guess that all are worth touching up.

The next category of body habits I want to dive into is body-position habits. Think about your day today. What percentage of the day were you sitting? What percentage were you standing? Walking? Lying down? Start considering 'static' vs 'active' positions as well. I will break it down for you. Let's say you have a desk job. Make an estimate of how many hours of the workday you are sitting vs standing vs walking. If you are (mostly) in one body-position, such as typing or writing or answering phones, etc. then it would go under 'static' sitting. If you take a bike ride after work, this would be 'active' sitting. Consider your whole day and put an estimated amount of time for each basic position: Sitting, Standing, Walking, Lying down (include both active and static activities for each). Then from each basic position category, get a rough estimate of how much is active vs static in that position. This is good information for later. If any of this is confusing, just do the overall sitting/standing/

walking/lying down estimates and leave it at that. It will give you an idea of what percentage of each day you are in each position. Then we can look even more specifically at what your body habits are like in certain positions.

Once you start really thinking about it in a 24-hour period, you can get an overall idea of what your body is actually doing on your average day. If your days are drastically different day-to-day, then you can look at an average workday vs a day-off day. Or, just do your best. All I can ask! Write down your overall hours (or percentage) for each basic position. Factor in sleep-time as well for lying down.

Now, we will add one more category to the mix. We will call this the Repetitive Movement category. For ease, we will just keep it to bigger-motion activities such as bending forward or reaching overhead, as opposed to fine motor repetition such as typing. There will be some overlap from your first list/calculation, so don't worry about that. Just write down total time in a day that involves some kind of repetitive motion. An example would be if you worked in a bookstore and spent 2 hours per shift shelving books (whether that is bending down towards the floor somewhat repetitively for lower shelves or boxes, or it is reaching up/overhead while standing with a straight back). Try to separate bending forward time and overhead reaching time. Don't get bogged down separating, but just make an estimate for each.

I will give you another example, just to help you out in categorizing. If you garden and you spend it mostly sitting with some motion but mostly static for chunks of time, just consider it sitting. If you work in a garden center and are bending over to get items and stock them, you can put that time under STANDING and also put that time under REPETITIVE MOTION (bending, or whatever sounds closest to the overall motion). If in doubt, just do your best. Don't worry about overlap, etc. We are just information gathering to get an overall sense of your average day.

The next body habit to dissect is one you are surely familiar with... POSTURE! The corrections are in the details of course, but the first step is just to notice. In each of the body position categories above (sitting, standing, walking, lying down, repetitive motion), consider your posture while you are in those positions. Yes, this includes sleep positioning!

If we look at sitting, and let's say you have a desk job of some sort (or are a professional chess player, or watch a lot of TV, or whatever your situation is)... notice what position your lower back tends to be in. Do you slump/round your back, or do you consciously sit up with a straight lower back? What position are your shoulders in? Are they rounded forward, or do you keep them slightly back more in line with your ears? Or, do you tend to raise them up TOWARDS your ears? A lot of people do this and have no idea they are doing it! Talk about neck-muscle overload! Next think about your head/chin position. Do you tend to jut your chin forward or keep it back? Do you tend to 'lead' with your head towards your computer screen, or do you keep your head from creeping towards whatever you are working on? Just start paying attention to what your postural habits are currently. Pssst: just noticing these things can be a lot like food journaling in that you start self-correcting just by clueing into what you're doing.

When you are standing, do you tend to rest your weight on one particular foot? Do you feel like you are in a relatively symmetrical and straight standing position? What about as you fatigue? This can give you some big clues. Notice if you tend to lock your knees. Notice if you tend to do what's called 'hip drop.' This would be having your weight towards one leg (so you have more pressure on one of your feet), while your hip on the OPPOSITE side 'drops' or relaxes downward. It is a 'relaxed' position for a lot of people while standing. I am describing the 'drop' this way, so that you can picture what I mean, but what is actually happening is you are relaxing the outer hip muscle on the STANCE leg (same side that you are putting more weight).

I bring the 'hip drop' up now for several reasons. It is very common AND most people don't know they are doing it. It is worth noticing on yourself. It weakens the outer hip muscle (gluteus medius if you like knowing that sort of thing) on the stance side AND is not awesome for your hip/lower back! It can also cause strain further down the chain (knees/feet). And that is just in standing. Weakness, or poor alignment from this weakness, can be a much bigger problem with 'active' movements such as walking (and even more so, running). So, all in all, worth a notice!

Much like locking your knees back, you can start to rid yourself of the habit just by knowing you are doing it. If you lock your knees, just slightly 'unlock' them when you do notice. If you tend to hip-drop, just try to avoid the 'sag' position. This will keep the hip muscle engaged (and keep it stronger), instead of letting yourself hang out in poor alignment for your back/hip. When you 'unlock' your knees, you are now letting your quadriceps muscles (front of your thighs) engage instead of putting strain on your knee, as well as improving alignment down the chain.

Of course, there are ways to actively strengthen your quadriceps and gluteus medius as well, which is excellent (I would say one of the weakest and most overlooked muscles is the gluteus medius). In 17 years of treating patients, I only tested 3 people who had full strength in this muscle!! So, let's just say I spent a lot of time with people working on their GM!

As for the rest of the postural habits, just pay attention to any other asymmetrical positions your body tends to move into while you are relatively still. Some people don't realize they lean or twist to one side while sitting or standing. Any repetitive or prolonged bending or twisting can be a problem over time, and speaking of time, it is cumulative when it comes to what it can do to your body. If you can do something very asymmetrical and feel like it is no big deal because you don't have pain…just a heads-up that it may be on its way. Better to reduce or balance out the additive poor positions or repetitive motions before it 'catches up with you.'

One of the most common pain conditions is lower back pain. If you have ever had an 'episode' of back pain, you know what I am talking about. It can really put a damper on your plans! Most lower back pain is from poor posture or repetitive motions such as forward bending. There are plenty of single-incident injuries of course, but I just wanted to let you know most is actually from cumulative position or action over time. So, let's get a good handle on what your body tends to do, so you can start to correct and reduce these common problems! For right now, just think of your spine as a relatively straight line (it has curves, but for simplicity for the moment, think about it as straight). If your body puts 'its weight' forward or backward or to one side, causing your spine to bend forward, or significantly backward, or into a sidebend position… it is worth paying attention to this.

In terms of your head/neck/shoulder position, think of your head as 'in line' with your body. If your head wants to sit well forward of what you picture as a straight line down your spine, then take notice and gently try to reduce that 'forward head' position. If you tend to 'jut' your chin forward (which means your neck is in an overly curved spine position), think of keeping a 'long neck.' Or, think of a slight 'chin tuck.' No one likes this idea, because they feel it gives them a 'double chin,' but, just correct slightly! Know that whatever your body is USED to doing is its current baseline, so anything you notice and want to change…be very gradual and gentle and subtle at first. If you try to all of a sudden change your body position/endurance, etc., your body can freak out just as if you over-trained at the gym.

Here is where I will throw in some obvious, but necessary, comments. Nothing you do when you start making adjustments that are new for your body should be painful or overly stressful. Everything I am talking about is part of a generalized habit change method that is beneficial for most people. However, if you have a medical condition, or have any pain, you should consult a specialist to address this. Since I am not individualizing any of these habit changes, keep in mind you should only do what you are comfortable with. I am simply giving you tips on very common body habits that you might need some reminders to pay attention to! This applies to everything in this book! Ok, good.

My next question for you: Are you abdominally aware? I don't mean do you notice abs on other people (I mean, do your thing) … but do you 'use' your own abs while going about your day? Now, they will naturally do certain things for you, which is great! And yes, you DO have abs… for those of you wondering if they are there. I want to remind you that: 1) you have them and 2) you can use them to HELP you! I will try to keep it simple here.

You have upper abs, lower abs, and obliques. Yes, you DO! Even if you can't see them clearly. The great news is you have them. They are there to protect you, stabilize you, and all-around keep you from falling over a lot.

The particular muscle I want you to notice lives roughly just below your waistline. Think belly button and below. Don't think about your 'crunch' muscles or your 'sit up' muscles (upper abs). Don't think rotational muscles (obliques). Just think about the muscle that essentially draws your lower stomach 'in' or towards your spine. Yes, the one that lets you zip up your extra…fitted… jeans. Side bonus, when strong, they also give you a more toned 'waistline.' Ok, now that we all know what we are talking about, those.

Your lower abs are your friend! Notice them! They stabilize your spine, protect your lower back, and are very important for optimal physical function from the rest of your body. If you think about it, it's your center. If it is strong (and active), it stabilizes your back/pelvis/hips, which in turn allows everything 'up' the chain and 'down' the chain to operate from a stable/solid center-point.

To activate them, all you have to do is very slightly draw 'in' your lower stomach, much like if you were putting on those aforementioned jeans. However, maybe not as aggressively as you might have for the jeans. Just see if you can draw them in slowly, while not moving any other part of your body (including your lower back). Think belly towards the spine, not crunch or curl. Subtle. Tiny, really. But huge for stability!

Also, remember to keep breathing while you contract your abs. You want to slowly draw in the stomach muscle, but you also want to avoid holding your breath. It takes a little concentration/ practice, but you want to train it this way so that when you start using it during other activities you are still breathing normally!

I am setting the stage here for what will become foundational body habits for the rest of your amazing life. Let your abs be a part of the fun! All the things we talk about I personally believe are some of the best things you can do for yourself, no matter what your activities or fitness routines entail. These are part of the foundation. Then, whatever else you do can complement, or build on, your solid foundation. They will also serve to protect you from injuries that you can hopefully avoid, because you are already taking care of yourself. You are ahead of the game! Creating a 'higher' baseline for yourself also gives you a higher threshold for all the other varied and less frequent activities you may get into, whether you are a weekend warrior or are going after your bucket list adventures! It allows you to more safely take on new, bigger challenges or adventures. It gives you a much better chance of avoiding all the pesky injuries and inflammatory conditions that like to show up more often as we age.

For example, you decide to go on a moderate hike. You think, I feel fine, this will be great! Never mind that you haven't walked

7 miles, or even close, in a very long while. You go, it's awesome, except that you end up with heel pain for the next 6 months that annoys the hell out of you and stops you from doing even your normal 'easy' activities. Now, hopefully this never happens to you. I am just saying… some version of this happens to A LOT of people. Or, you finally get to go to Europe, and you start walking all around the beautiful cities and half way through your trip, uggghhhhhh… walking is PAINFUL! I know so many people who have had trips go sadly VERY sedentary. All I am saying here is, get your baseline game up a notch so you can do your thing!

I am sure you have heard the phrase 'use it or lose it.' Well, it is quite appropriate to expand on here! Because HERE is where I want to talk about walking. Yep. Plain ol' walking. If you do one thing for yourself for the rest of your life (I shouldn't say that… because… there are a few other 'one' things), BUT, if you do one thing for the rest of your life, when it comes to baseline exercise… take a walk every day. Here are the parameters. Walk, comfortable speed, comfortable and supportive shoes, continuously, for 20-30 min, every day. That's it. That's the big secret!

If you walk 30 minutes, continuously, as your baseline 'normal' daily activity, you won't just wake up one day and realize you can't walk for 30 minutes. Now, understand I am talking about the use-it-and-you-won't-lose-it concept. Yes, you could have an injury or medical condition or inflammatory situation that puts you off this habit until you are recovered. Yes. What I am talking about is simple. You won't lose the basic body-conditioned ability to walk for 30 minutes non-stop, as long as you keep it going (barring other medical issues). Let me put it this way…after treating patients for

17 years, I discovered that the people who were still kickin' it and very active well into their 80s and 90s (yep, 90s!) all had this in common. So, needless to say, I took notice!

I always asked every patient about their daily routines and exercise habits, and I noticed that those that made it a priority to make sure they took a walk FOR exercise (not just stop and go, or while working, etc.) definitely seemed to be healthier and more resilient overall. This is just my take-away and something I feel strongly about, in terms of passing along to all of you. The benefits of a walk every day are numerous, and I could list a lot of reasons I do it. There is no doubt it is good for blood flow, general muscle strength/endurance (yes, just walking), etc., but it is also a time for you to disconnect from all the many things that aren't so healthy in your daily life. If you sit a lot, you want to counter that activity with a walk anyway. If you are stressed, you want to counter that with blood flow and you-time. And even more effective is finding a place you can walk that is actually pleasant to you and your senses! Nature, of course, is the best! But if you don't have a pleasant option outside, to give you the bonus of fresh air and stress-reducing surroundings, then just do that part when you DO have the option. Personally, every time I have moved (which has been A LOT), one of my first considerations is having a good walk option nearby. But, that's just me. I obviously put it high on the priority list!

I think this is understood, but I do realize that there are some days it just doesn't happen. Or, you get injured and have to gradually build it back in. But that's kind of the point. It is part of your 'normal' day, so if you don't do it some days or you have to stop temporarily, it is not a detriment at all. You just get back to it when it is appropriate. Also, if you are not used to walking that long AT ALL, then remember to just gradually build your routine (starting with 15 minutes, or whatever is pain-free and good for you). It would be pointless to give yourself plantar fasciitis (heel pain) in the process! So, use whatever is your current baseline, what you know your body is happy with, then slowly build that up over time until you are happy and used to 20-30 minutes per day.

Here is a good moment to mention purging some things. We only have so many minutes in a day. So, if you are starting to think about adding new things (like a 30 min walk), you may want to also start thinking about activities you can reduce/purge that are not serving you so well. I am not here to judge how you spend your time - it's your time! You will prioritize what you feel is best for you. I am just saying maybe you could find 10 minutes of the day that you … oh, I don't know, unintentionally find yourself checking Facebook or Instaface or whatever else is your thing… and use that towards a walk instead? Oh, and a buzzkill for those of you already strategizing walking WHILE being on Instaface…ideally, your head/neck/body is in a straight walking-to-walk position! Sorry. Just helping your neck out.

Ok, one more EASY habit for you! Breathe. There is an interesting thing that happens when we are busy, stressed, or well, for many, just living life…we tend to shallow breathe. It's kind of like we forget to really breathe! Luckily, as we talked about earlier in the book, our brain takes care of making sure we do breathe, without having to think about it. But, it's a great habit to take in bigger breaths on/off throughout the day. I don't mean go around gasping in people's faces - not cool! When you shallow breathe or chronic-stress breathe, the accessory muscles in the neck often over-work. This adds to neck tightness and tension that you probably already have anyway! Try just the starter-habit of just 5 deep breaths one time per day. Yes! That's it. Once that is a habit… you know the drill. Feel free to add reps or increase times per day you interrupt the busy stress-mode breathing you're so good at. Intentional breathing is a great habit to incorporate in your day.

We will revisit the walking-is-good-for-you and breathing-is-good-for-you routine when we combine all your body habits together in a more comprehensive way, but I couldn't resist getting those to you now! Walk. Breathe. Every day. My work here is done! Well, I suppose that would be a bit book-cut-short of me, so maybe more accurately… A great start! My work continues! Not here. In Chapter 5. When you're ready…

Tips:

Take Inventory on:

1. **Food Habits**
2. **Hydration Habits**
3. **Sleep Habits**
4. **Body Position Habits**
5. **Repetitive Motion Habits**
6. **Postural/asymmetrical Habits**
7. **Abdominal stabilization Habits**
8. **Walking Habits**
9. **Breathing Habits**

CHAPTER 5

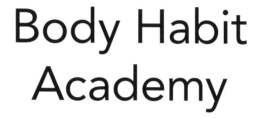

Body Habit Academy

Welcome to Body Habit Academy! Now that we have gotten a good idea of what our body baseline habits are currently, we want to get into ways we can establish and re-set a new (and improved) baseline for ourselves. This is not easy to do because our bodies (and minds) are accustomed to our current habits. So, consider it a challenge to yourself to make some habit changes that can help serve you better, for the rest of your life. Once you have overcome the initial hurdle of change (Ahhhh!!!!), your bodies and minds will settle into the simple, yet effective, new baseline habits. Then, your subconscious will also assist you in these new routines!

For some of you these ideas/changes will be relatively easy, in theory, to incorporate into your lives. You may already do some pieces of these things and you are just modifying or adding to an already established habit. In these cases, you can use whatever system/cues you already have to make the new habits happen. You are just changing the details of the habit itself. For others, all of these habits are brand new. This is a bit more challenging in that you will need to find cues/triggers to remind yourself to do ALL of these things. In either case, we are using all the help we can get from our own mind/creativity/current routines in any way we can to make the transitions as smooth as possible!

Keep in mind a few things while you are working on incorporating new habits 1) The WHY you are doing them i.e., your health and well-being! 2) The longer you stick to it/consciously work at it, the MUCH easier it gets over time i.e., after 3 weeks of hardcore conscious tactics! 3) Your body will also adjust over time and make physical changes (along with your brain) to make it all that much easier i.e., 3 months! 4) You. Are. In. Control. Be your own habit-change boss and make it happen!

Ok. POSTURE! Get this. Your body adapts to whatever position you are in the most. What I mean by this is your muscles literally change length to match prolonged positions you adopt. For instance, if you sit a lot, your hamstrings (back of your legs between your butt and your knees) shorten and tighten because sitting with knees bent is a 'short' position for your hamstring muscles. The same idea applies to your hip flexors (the front of your hips) because sitting is also a 'short' position for these guys. This does not just apply to the big lower body muscles. If you sit with your shoulders relaxed (gravity!) forward, the muscles on the front side of your shoulders/chest also shorten.

Now, consider the physics of all of this. If your shoulders are rounded forward and the front side muscles shorten... well, then the muscles opposite them (back side of your shoulders and upper back) have to lengthen to allow this position as well. When the muscles lengthen beyond their optimal length, they also weaken! So... you get short and tight in certain muscle groups and long and weaker in opposite muscles groups. Double whammy! All of this creates muscle imbalances that throw off muscle length/strength, joint dynamics (forces going through your joints differently/stressfully), and overuse/compensation strategies that your body uses to attempt to battle the poor alignment/overuse/imbalance. I am saying all this so you get that your body is made up of a bunch of pulley systems and physics problems! If you are imbalanced, it throws off all the desired angles and forces that your body works at its best! Over time, these forces cause strain on certain areas and create wear and tear, stress, inflammation, and the list goes on. So… it is to your HUGE advantage, especially as we age, to get things lined up as best as you can to make your body as happy and smoothly working as possible! Enter… ME! I want this for you.

Let's get into some solutions. Problems always want solutions, we just have to find them, be open to do them, and… yes… those same two words… do them. That's the hard part. And please keep in mind, as I have said before, these are all suggestions for those that do not have medical conditions, etc. that do not like any change, even 'good' change. If you have any issues with anything I suggest, consult your doctor/clinician first.

90% of people have some episode of lower back pain at some point in their lives. For some, it is acute and does not return, but for many, it does return or become chronic/episodic. In most of these cases, the cause is not one incident, but a cumulative effect of strain/stress/poor positioning over time. This is why posture/alignment is so important to understand/be aware of. I am sure you know you should 'sit up straight.' But, how much attention do you actually pay to this on a daily basis? Hopefully you are already working on it, at least somewhat.

If your lower back is 'slumped,' not only does it add to improper alignment of your spine and back muscles, but it does two other things 1) it puts the rest of your upper body into gravity-wins-hard position because now you are already in a forward head/forward shoulders position and 2) it puts significant pressure on the front side of your lumbar discs. Let me go into this a little more.

Picture the discs in your lower back as little cushions between each of the vertebra in your spine. They serve as shock absorbers up and down the spine. The discs (cushions) have a fibrous outer layer, but the center is more jelly-like. So, this means the 'stuffing' in those cushions can squish forward or backwards or side to side, depending on where the pressure is coming from. If your spine is in a good straight line overall, the stuffing is mostly centered. However, if you bend forward (or slouch in sitting), then there is much more pressure concentrated on the front of the cushion. You are now squishing the stuffing towards the back of the cushion, which is towards your back (and also the nerves that hang out back there). This is where 'bulging discs' come from. And if you are really unlucky and there is enough pressure to bust the stuffing out the back side of the cushion's outer layer, then you have a herniated disc. Ouch. Bigtime.

It is not just the discs we want to take care of. When you slouch (or lose the natural inward curve of your lower back and create the OPPOSITE curve in your lower back), you are also putting your lower back muscles in a poor 'resting' position. Over time, your lower back may eventually rebel against this poor position and scream at you in the form of back spasms, 'going out on you,' and all kinds of other tantrums. In short, I highly recommend sitting up straight! This does not mean you can never relax in your favorite chair or relax your lower back. Just remember the whole percentage of the day/life thing! And here is where your list of positions/number of hours in a day comes into play. It is not just sitting for long periods; it is also cumulative for all activities that you may be in a rounded-back position. So, it is not that you have to ALWAYS have your back straight, it is just a change in percentage you want. In fact, it is good to let your back relax, it is just not good to adopt a prolonged position (or habit) of slouching.

Now I am going to get more specific. I mentioned that 'sit up straight' part, because overall this is the easiest way to think about it (and if that is all that makes sense to you, just go with that). BUT, the best change is in the details, if you are up for the details! Your lower back naturally has a slight 'inward' curve (think convex, if you are looking at someone's lower back) just above the tailbone. This amount of curve can vary depending on the person, but generally it is slightly curved 'in.'

When you stand and place your hand flat, just above your tailbone (hey, this is good - you should stand anyway for a short bit to break up the sitting and reading!), you can feel a slight inward curve. Consider that your natural curve that you want to mimic while sitting unsupported. As soon as you sit, you will lose this curve (gravity combined with the least amount of work possible by your muscles!) unless you actively 'put' it there. It is no mystery why we slouch - energy conservation! Your lower back muscles have to work to support your spine in a straight back position. This is also why any changes you make should be gradual/intermittent/kind to your poor untrained back muscles!

Now, if you are sitting on your couch or comfy chair and are starting to want to burn this book because you don't want to have to sit up straight and never enjoy your couch, don't fret (or set anything on fire). When you are sitting 'supported,' just keep in mind that anything that reduces the REVERSE of that curve is helpful. I have a habit for you. When you go to relax on your couch, just throw a comfy couch pillow behind your lower back to help reduce the extra-rounded position that many couches suck you into. BUT, when you are sitting, say, at your desk or waiting for a bus, unsupported, then think about trying to re-create the SLIGHT inward curve that is natural for your lower back. This is a good start - more to come.

I think it's best to think of the posture/rounded back problem as something you make gradual and small changes that are reasonable, and you can control. There are going to be LOTS of times you either can't control a poor position or don't remember to, so we need habits to at least reduce those parts of the equation that you can control. Remember, it is additive, so you are just subtracting a bit. Let's start with the obvious first... GET UP! If you have a desk job or hobby or passion that requires sitting... 1) Get up as often as you can that is reasonable for your situation 2) Correct your posture (!) while you do have to maintain the seated position. Like I said, starting with the obvious. Obvious, yet definitely not put into action by most people in their daily lives. It is quite difficult to make this happen, unless you 'put your mind to it.' So, first, we want to tackle the 'slump' habit. Step one: Notice. Pay attention. Step two: Create a cue/trigger for a correction. More to come on that. But, just like the food journaling and the hip dropping, you will start to correct once you actually pay attention to what you are doing/not doing in the first place.

By the way, when I say 'slump,' I don't just mean extreme slouching. A lot of people say 'no, I sit up straight - I don't slump.' But, remember that a 'slouch' has variations and what we are paying attention to is how much curve reversal you have going on. So, you may be ahead of the slump game by making sure you don't extreme-slump (good!!), but you may not realize you still reverse your (slight) curve in your lower back most of the time while sitting. Oh... I should also say... I keep saying SLIGHT, because you do not want to OVER correct or exaggerate your natural curve. If you are unsure, just think 'straight' spine instead. At the very least, you will not be allowing it into a concave (rounded) position. Have I beat you over the head with this? Not my intention! But, it is a very commonly missed, very basic, habit change that can do amazing things for you in terms of the happy-body-later category. The weird thing about it is that you will never actually KNOW you prevented things... because, well, you prevented them. But, I can tell you from experience in both my career and myself personally, it is worth the change/work. Just think of your cute little cushions in there celebrating the relief after all that squishing that's been going on.

Now, for strategy. Since you need to be mindful of not overdoing any new position or muscle work to avoid a negative body reaction to change (yep, the body is just as freaked out by change, even if it is GOOD change, as a lot of people are in general), you need to start small and then build on it. Let's say you have a desk job (or hobby, etc.), and you sit 6 hours/day overall (consult your list). Habit #1: Set an alarm (or whatever alerts you consistently, like a Katie that points at you) every hour that alerts you to get up. Even if all you do is stand and walk around in your tiny office or workspace for 20 seconds. Or, you can just simply stand and 'shake it out.' Or, you can stand and gently lean backwards, in the opposite direction of bending forward, slowly a few times. Or, you can just stand up. The point here is GET UP, even if brief.

On to Habit #2: While you are sitting during that hour, try to occasionally self-correct your back position. Just start with the idea of self-correction as you think of it. You will inconsistently remember/correct and then forget/relax, and this is ok. This primes your lower back that change is coming! Ok, so now you get up and twirl, or gently lean backwards in standing, or do your best 20-second dance... whatever gets you up every hour AND you intermittently self-correct your posture as noticed. Try this for a week to start the change. Once you know how much you are actually catching yourself and how your back is reacting to the change, you can then put into place a more specific 'training' habit. Now you need the alarm/arm-pointing friend/computer-generated reminder/whatever-cues-you-CONSISTENTLY trigger for sitting up straight. Yes, it is highly annoying at first! You could try a post-it or something less annoying, but then... you are less likely to be yanked out of your running-on-autopilot brain to make the necessary changes so that sitting up straight becomes your NEW running-on-autopilot habit. It takes persistence and consistency, but eventually, you will notice when you DON'T sit up straight. In fact, you may start to 'feel' the little cushions asking for some help once you become more in tune with what a pressured back feels like vs an 'unsquished' position.

I am not saying you can actually feel your discs per se, but you will start to become much more aware of what a 'good' spinal position feels like and WANT it. It is just fatiguing, because it takes muscle work. Hence, why you need to gradually train them to do this important job. You can/should only do what your back tolerates, so go easy and gradually on how often you ask them to kick in and help. Everything is baseline and build, especially when the habit is a body position/muscle work change. You need to give 'breaks' on anything that feels like stress/strain. Give it time to train and adjust, just like any new exercise or workout or sport. This is the highly non-competitive sport of Posture!

Foundation building here. Ok, once you start to have the lower back habit taking hold, now add in the shoulders/head position part! The great news is that as you correct the lower back position, everything up the chain follows suit naturally. So, once your body is used to a straighter back position, you can add the more subtle details up the chain.

If your lower back is in a good, straight position, then just add a slight 'shoulders back' correction. Think about just barely squeezing the muscles between your shoulder blades (these muscles pull your shoulders back). Remember, THIS IS SUBTLE. If you try to crank your shoulders back and fully squeeze your shoulder blades when your body is used to 'forward shoulders,' you will surely hate me. Please don't hate me! Just think 'shoulders slightly back.' Then work this habit in with the same cue you have for lower back correction. Intermittent upper back strengthening/ postural strengthening is what is going on here. So, much like the lower back muscles, you can allow them to relax when fatigued or forgotten at first. Later, you can increase the frequency of your reminder cue.

Ok, two postural corrections down, one to go! Chin/head/ neck position is next. If you didn't get my SUBTLE reminder before, you should REALLY pay attention to it now. Correcting your head/ neck position is tricky for some people. The biggest thing is to do this as subtly as possible and then gradually correct more. But, here is the deal. We are talking about the 'chin tuck' correction that I mentioned earlier. Think about your neck being in a 'long' position or think 'tiny double chin.' I know! But, this will make you less likely to overdo it at least! Basically, you are just making sure your head is not trying to creep forward of your body (forward head). So, for a lot of people, the best verbal description is to think about 'tucking' your chin straight back, in the direction of making a double chin. Ha. I just feel your discontent with this unflattering thought. SUBTLE.

Once you feel the difference in your neck position (you are reducing the squish in your neck cushions and getting your poor neck muscles on the back of your neck out of a short position when you correct this), you will be able to get the notion of a 'longer' neck when you chin tuck. At the very least, just notice if you tend to lead with your head or jut your head/chin forward. Try to reduce the amount of 'forward head' position as much as feels ok to you.

By the way, lengthening these muscles at the back of your neck also helps to reduce muscle-induced headaches. These muscles attach to the base of your skull, and when short/in a prolonged 'short' position, they can create headache pain over time. Prevention for muscle-induced headaches includes this 'chin tuck' technique. So, all the more reason to do it!

Ok. Now you have the three basic sitting posture habits you are putting into place, to re-set your overall posture position: 1) Lower back 'straight' or slight inward curve 2) Shoulders slightly back 3) Head/chin slightly back. This position allows your whole spine to have as close to the natural (and protective) curves that you (hopefully) have when you stand. A lot of people still have some forward head and forward shoulders in standing as well, it is just that they are generally more pronounced while sitting due to the lower back relaxing/slouching in sitting. So, certainly feel free to continue the corrections for shoulders/neck in standing/walking later as you get used to it.

Posture:

1) **Lower back straight**
2) **Shoulders slightly back**
3) **Chin/head slightly back**

Here are a few extra tips when it comes to postural correction change. If you know you will be sitting for more than 15-20 minutes, or will be regularly in one particular spot/workspace, etc., assist your posture position by making sure whatever you are working on is as close to you as possible. If you have to reach out in front of you, then you are adding more work from your back side muscle groups (lower back, upper back, neck) to counter the reach/weight of your arms forward. The further your arms are out in front, away from your body, the more muscle work it takes for your postural muscles to stabilize you.

You are already working hard enough trying to correct your posture, without the added work to counter the weight of your arms. So, it is best to have your keyboard as close to you as possible, to allow your arms to be closer to your body (upper arms in line with your sides). If you are reaching for the phone or things on your desk a lot, just try to bring those items closer to you. If you add up all the reaching or prolonged arms-out-in-front-of-you time during the day/week/month/years, it adds to the postural challenge as well as neck/upper back strain.

There are many more specific ergonomic adjustments you can make, but for the sake of simplicity here, just remember that what matters most is the actual position your body is in. You could have the most expensive ergonomic chair and keyboard set-up (which can be great help!), but if you don't make sure to make the active body-position changes a habit, you will still have the same issues.

Now we move on to repetitive motion habits. You now know the most protective position for your spine/body overall. We can apply that same position during 'active' motions, it just takes some concentration at first. If your day requires certain activities that mean repetitive bending or lifting or reaching (see your list of repetitive motion), your best protection against injury or 'wear and tear' problems is to apply the same 'set' position for your spine as best as you can.

If you have to bend forward or lift, remember the natural inward curve of your spine you have when you are upright. To keep this position for your spine, you need to make the bend come from your hips instead of your lower back. This is key! The hips were meant to bend, but your lower back (and your cute little discs) are no longer protected once you bend your back. So, think 'butt out' when you bend forward or lift. Yep, stick your butt out. Not aggressively! It's just a helpful mental cue to be able to keep the back straight while bending at the hips.

Think about how toddlers tend to pick up things from the

ground when they are first learning to do this from a standing position. They square up and then bend their knees and hips (and stick their butt out) while they steady themselves to bend forward. So, it seems we know what to do instinctively… and then let it all go as we get older! Granted, part of this technique when we are first learning to use our bodies, is to avoid falling on our heads when we lean forward… a lesson in counterbalance! But, we also tend to bend from our hips instead of rounding our back to bend over. Better balance AND better form - well done tiny humans!

Back to the repetitive motion category. So, you keep your back straight (inwardly curved) when you bend forward or lift. Now, add the shoulders/head 'set' position to the mix. If you are lifting, first remember to keep the object as close to your body as possible, to reduce extra strain to counter the arms-out position (but now with weight, so exponentially greater strain). Next, remember the shoulders slightly back/chin slightly back protection position while you lift/carry, reach, etc. There are situations when this is very difficult, but if you get in the habit of 'setting' those muscles/positions, you will at least reduce the cumulative effect/strain over time. This is a numbers game: reduce the percentage of 'bad habit' moments and increase the percentage of 'good habit' moments. You are not looking for perfection. That's just stressful itself! You are reducing the chances of the eventual 'breaking point' for repetitive stress injuries for lower back, neck, and shoulders just by putting these new set-position habits in place. Lower back pain, neck pain, and shoulder pain/strain/tears are unfortunately very common. The good news is that so many of them are quite preventable! If you have been able to avoid these so far in your life, a big congratulations! Let's keep it that way!

Speaking of added protection from injury... Abs, Abs, Abs!! I like to think of this section as Abdominal Intelligence 101. You already know where the muscle lives (lower stomach, belly button and below). And for those of you who like names, let me introduce you to Transverse Abdominis! We shall call her TA. You also already know how to activate your TA: remember the zipping up your favorite 'going out' jeans? Yes, so, you activate your TA by drawing your lower stomach towards your spine. Also, remember to think about only moving your lower stomach 'inward' without moving other parts of your body, including your lower back. Activated! Ok, so you know where it is, how to activate it, and what it does (protects your lower back, as well as being your center-stabilization point for the rest of your body). No big deal, just your lower back and the rest of your body.

Now all we have to do is teach you to actually USE it. The good news is that it will kick in on its own without conscious thought for certain counterbalance activities and daily movements. The bad news is that it is often quite INACTIVE otherwise, unless you have been training it/using it along the way. You can train it to work on cue FOR you, for added protection/stabilization. And like most habits, over time, it will start to kick in even more with less thought. On top of that, the stronger it is, the more it will do for you. All good things!

There are countless ways to incorporate TA activation with daily activities, but since I like efficiency, let's pick a cue that is already happening in your new habit routine. You can add it to your daily walk and consider it started! You can also link it to any other activity of your choice, but training it while you walk has extra benefits in that it SHOULD be working for you when you walk anyway. Most people have to actively think about it to get to going more consistently, so that is a good place to start.

My suggestion is that you think of it as ab-training at the beginning and end of your walk, for starters. When you start your walk (let's say for the first 1-2 minutes), gently activate the TA and hold for roughly 3-5 steps (or seconds, whatever short time period works for you) and then relax for the same (3-5 steps). You don't need to be exact by any means, you will get a feel for what works as comfortable repetitions. You could start with just the first couple minutes and last couple minutes of your 20-30 minute walk to get the habit going. As you get more used to what it feels like, as well as letting your body adjust to it, you can sprinkle in more rounds or just do intermittent reps here and there when you think about it in between.

Reminder: this should not change your overall back position or anything for that matter, but you may feel a slight change in how your hips feel in stride because you are now actually stabilizing your pelvis while your legs do their thing to walk. If you have tight hip flexors (front of your hips), you may feel even more difference in your natural stride. If you have REALLY tight hip flexors, you may find you need to reduce your stride distance a tiny bit to allow this adjustment. Either way, it should not feel like you are actively moving other parts of you in order to just activate the TA. If you do, reduce the aggressiveness of your contraction/activation. Go for SUBTLE. I have never typed that word so much in my life!

Once you get used to what if feels like to activate your lower abs, then add the habit with more cues, such as every time you change position. Not SUBTLE position changes (just felt like another one there), but big position changes like going from sit to/from stand, or lying down to getting up, etc. This is naturally when your TA is supposed to kick in anyway (again, it's here to protect your lower back and stabilize as you move your body), but for many, it is lacking or just plain inactive. The more you consciously activate, the smarter it gets! Over time, you will start to do it without thought, but my advice is to keep the habit going actively even if your body starts to take over for you. It is just more protection and more strength all around. This comes into play when you do things that aren't so 'healthy' for you such as repetitive heavy lifting, twisting, and countless other life-activities that stress the back. If your lower abs are 'set,' your body is able to handle more strain, much like the rest of the 'set' positions I've mentioned so far.

When you get really good (and efficient, if that's your thing), you can add it to other daily activities such as brushing your teeth (yes, I still like that you brush your teeth) or doing the dishes or walking to your car or anything else that happens regularly and intermittently. The TA is gloriously protective AND toning, so there's that extra nugget, too! Eventually, the TA activation along with your 'set' position for your posture/spine, will serve you wonderfully during all things exercise/life! But first, you just need to work on making it a habit with one aspect of daily life. Don't overwhelm yourself. Start small. And be consistent.

Ok, now let's get into countermeasures. You now know what position you are trying to put yourself into (a better one, yes). But, for all the times you are not necessarily successful at that, we have counter-actions we can do to help balance it out a bit. If you sit a lot (this includes active sitting like biking), ideally, you do counter motions to sitting 1-2x/day. Sitting involves the back wanting to go into 'bend' position. So, the countermeasure habit for bending (or flexion) is extension (gently moving your back into the opposite direction).

You can introduce an extension movement for your back in standing (mentioned earlier, just slowly leaning backwards a little bit, in standing) or lying down. The lying down version would be lying on your stomach and using your arms to gently lift your upper body/chest up, while relaxing your lower back/legs/butt. You would just allow your lower back, etc. to sag/relax on the floor, so that you are getting a gentle reversal of the forward bend position of your spine. Don't forget the this-applies-to-healthy-backs-with-no-condition-that-does-not-warrant-extension thing.

For me personally, 3-5 reps, slowly, either standing or lying down works great as a countermeasure for 'poor' sitting positions at times during the day/night. It also just feels awesome to get a nice stretch. Even if you are posture-conscious, just think of it as countering the rounded-back position that happens when you relax in your chair or couch. Since flexion (forward bend) is a much more common repetitive motion for the average person then extension (backward bending), it is a good general stretch for many people. There are certain back conditions that extension is not a good thing, so consult your doctor or clinician if you have a medical condition of this kind.

Countermeasures can also include general stretches for overworked, repetitively-used muscles, or muscles in the 'short' position. For instance, for prolonged sitting, this would include hamstrings and hip flexors. If you start walking more (ahem), then you should also start stretching your calves more. With more walking comes more calf use (as well as other muscles, of course). The lower body muscles I make sure to include in my daily routine are 1) calves 2) hip flexors 3) hamstrings 4) gluts/butt muscles. I have a very specific stretching routine that works for me. I target the chronically tight/overworked muscle groups, as well as the ones that cause the most common inflammatory conditions.

I would happily share all my specifics with any of you, if we ever meet! But for the purposes of this book, I just want to at least spur you to consider a general stretching routine (even if you do yoga), that takes care of the most common muscle imbalance issues that crop up with cumulative activities/prolonged positions such as the ones above. Stretching helps counter what muscles you use the most, or what muscles get put in the short position the most. If you walk a lot, consider calves, hip flexors, hamstrings, and piriformis (butt/hip muscle). If you sit a lot, consider hamstrings, hip flexors, and piriformis. Then you can add other muscles that are particularly tight on you, including neck/shoulders, etc.

Your routine can vary depending on your activities/sports/work-outs/job/hobbies, etc., but when it comes to general prevention and countermeasures, these are some of the big areas to focus on. Whatever stretch routine you start with, make it a habit! Even if it is just your tightest two muscle groups. Since you are walking regularly, make sure to include your calves! You can start with a gentle 20-30 second stretch, 1-2 times on each muscle. Just so you know, there are two different types of 'static' stretching. If a muscle is actually SHORT (meaning, it has adapted to a short length due to being in a position over time), you would want to do a 20-30 second hold, 3 times, 2x/day in order to try to change the actual length of the muscle back to its optimal length. If your muscles are just tight, meaning stiff (but have not lost physical length overall), then generally, you can just do 1-2 rounds at 20-30 seconds to make sure they do not gradually shorten. Either way, a good start when it comes to a stretching habit, is to pick a couple muscles to do a general 'tightness' stretch as explained above.

It is good to understand that when a muscle is tight or short, it will change the mechanics of the body to account for that tension/length. Over time, it can create an imbalance in the body system overall (because, it's all connected)! It's just physics, really. Have you ever seen a person at the gym that looks like they are hugging an invisible bear? No? Well, it looks like they are hugging an invisible bear. At least to me. Their chest muscles are shorter (and stronger) than their opposite, upper back muscles, so their arms/shoulders are forward. As in, this is their 'relaxed' position! Their biceps are stronger (shorter) than the opposite (triceps) muscles, so their elbows are bent in a 'relaxed' position. So, if they are standing there… the only thing missing is an adorably large (and hopefully very friendly) bear in their inviting arms. Side note: you might have guessed that I just try not to look around when I am in the gym, to avoid calculating all the muscle imbalance (and possible wildlife) around me.

Muscle imbalance can be very mild and not-too-big-a-deal, which everyone has to some extent. We can't be perfect. That would be boring! However, if you sit in a position with forward shoulders, forward head, and rounded back for years, eventually your body adapts to that position as your 'resting' position. Muscles tighten/shorten, and the opposite muscles lengthen (and weaken), until it's your new 'normal.' If you take it even longer (age and cumulative effects coming into play), this is how some of the older population ends up stooped over and 'forward' all over! Of course, there are medical conditions that cause this as well, but for many, it is just gravity and muscle imbalance at play. Battle it. And battle it now, not after years of it make it even harder to reverse/ correct. For some, once it has adopted this position long enough, it is 'solidified' in ways that make it unsafe to try to correct.

For those of us who are lucky enough to not have a medical condition that stops us from winning this battle, we should take advantage of our ability to create habits now that give us the best shot at being upright and walking happily well into our forever-years. On that note, let's recap your 10 new daily body habits! Yippee!

Tips:

1) Walk (non-stop 20-30 min, in good walking shoes)
2) Breathe (5 deep breaths)
3) Unlock 'locked' knees
4) Avoid hip drop
5) Get up every hour (or more!)
6) Re-set posture position (try every 15 min)
   A) Back straight (slight inward curve)
   B) Shoulders slightly back
   C) Slight chin tuck
7) Use 'set' position for lifting/repetitive motion
8) Countermeasure for sitting (gentle extension 3-5 reps, 1-2x/day)
9) Lower Ab (TA) activation (with walking and/or position changes)

10) Stretch routine (20-30 sec, 1-3 reps) *calf muscles at very least!

Oh and ...

11) Go celebrate all your new habits!

CHAPTER 6

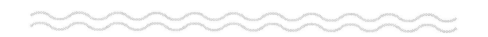

Physical Launch

Welcome back from your 10-habit celebration! Those new (or not-so-new) daily body habits are what I have found to be some of the most helpful and healthful very basic things you can do on a daily basis. There are many more and many variations of course, but I share these specifically because I truly believe they will help protect you and help you thrive, along with whatever else you may choose to do for yourself.

And now my friends, we have entered the Physical Launch Arena! I think of the 10 basic daily habits as just part of your everyday routine, like sleeping/eating/hydrating. Once you have that foundation in place, you can determine/set NEW goals that build on them, that propel you forward in fitness and general body health. So, here we go!

Think about what you want, when it comes to your body, and why. These kinds of goals can fall into 2 categories: 1) For your health/fitness/ideal weight in the sense of long-term achieve-and-maintain types of goals; 2) Single-event style goals such as walking/running a marathon/race, hiking a specific trail/mountain, etc. I will be mostly addressing Category #1 in this chapter because this is part of your foundation for life in general. Category #2 will be more in the realm of bucket-list-style goals, which we will get into in the next section of the book! Category #2 can build on #1, much like any other adventure or exciting challenge you decide to take on in your life. Of course, this is not to say you can't just go for Category 2 (you can do whatever you want - my book is not strong enough to stop you!), I am just speaking from the happier-body perspective in most of these cases. I am on your side!

Your goals are exactly that - yours. So, you can apply all of these things in ways that suit you and your happiness best. Whatever your goals for your body/health, there are ways to better serve you to actually 'be reliable' and do what you set out to do.

First, as described in Part I, you want to know WHAT the goal is exactly and WHY. Once you determine these two things (in earnest), you want to do some 'thought pattern' work (Part I coming at you hard!) regarding your goal. You want to be sure your underlying 'running thoughts' support your goal. This also means getting your subconscious beliefs/thoughts on the same page as your conscious desires. We want BOTH working towards your goal, not against.

Once you have the brain on board (happy, excited and believing in you), you can get into the PLAN mode. Here is where the points mentioned earlier kick in! You want your plan to 1) Be REAListic, step-wise, gradual, and healthy; 2) Be sustainable and maintainable; 3) Have a contingency plan, including excuse-crushers, work-arounds, modifications; 4) Have rewards/celebrations/rest/freedom built in!

Here's the thing. So many people want to lose weight or 'look good' or be more active or more fit, but any goal that involves the body CHANGING means it needs time to catch up and solidify a new baseline tolerance. Otherwise, especially as we age, we end up with changes we DON'T WANT like injured joints, inflammation, repetitive-use pain, muscle spasms, etc. We, instead, want our bodies to also be on board with our goals! This takes understanding, patience, adaptation, determination, and consistency. Here is the good news - you have all 5 of these things!

I feel sure of it! You just need a plan that includes them. You want your mind AND your body to be reliable in the process.

Sometimes we take for granted all that our bodies put up with… until they DON'T! Every step you take, literally, requires all kinds of actions and reactions in the body. The moment your heel strikes the ground, all the stabilizing muscles kick in, counterbalance muscles kick in, your cute little cushions in your back absorb the shock, your joints and internal structures in the joint join the shock-absorption team, and… that's just the initial heel-meets-ground impact moment! So, keep in mind that something as (for some) low-key as walking, adds up every step (or every rep).

Now remind yourself that the muscles that work the most get stronger (and tighter), and the opposite tend to weaken (in comparison). The bigger the imbalance, the more the bigger/stronger muscles take over in your general activities… which creates more imbalance and poor alignment. So, whatever muscles you start picking on more, just be aware you may want to increase your stretching routine for these tighter/stronger muscles to keep the length/tension imbalance from increasing. You may also want to think about adding some exercises for the 'opposite' muscle groups, so they are not so left out in the process. Put plainly, if you are trying to increase your overall fitness level and strength, you want a balanced routine.

Let's get more specific. If you are working out your upper body, make sure you include at least as much 'work' for your upper back ('rows' are a great general upper back and postural strengthening exercise!) as for the front side of you. If you work your biceps (front of your upper arms), then make sure you are also working your triceps (back side of your upper arms). Another thing to keep in mind is that certain muscle groups naturally work WAY harder all day long (anything you lift or carry tends to work the front-side muscles such as biceps/chest), which is why you want to focus on strengthening your opposite side (upper back, postural muscles, etc).

For most people, their 'back side' lower body is the 'tight side' and the 'back side' upper body is the 'weaker' side. For instance, often the hamstrings and calves are tighter than the quads and anterior tibs (yeah, I said 'tibs'). The anterior tibialis (pet name, tibs) is the muscle on the front of your lower leg that lifts your toes up to clear the ground, so you don't trip every step. Quite helpful! But, your calf muscles are what propel you forward, lift your heel up/push your toes into the ground, etc. Calves tend to have a tightness issue on most people, especially if you walk a lot. I say all of this just to remind you that some general stretching and some general counter-strengthening can save you from a lot of muscle imbalance/inflammation issues in the future. That, and I just wanted to say 'tibs.'

I think it is important to remember that what you are going for is a consistent and healthy fitness level that can serve you to be able to do all the other things you want to do in life. This is why it is helpful to think of it as gradually increasing your baseline exercise foundation until it becomes your new 'normal'. Everything else you choose to do (training for a specific event, trying a new sport, finding a new hobby, playing a new instrument, or being a weekend warrior in general) puts your body under a new version of stress. This doesn't have to be bad stress; it can just be muscle-building stress. That is how we build muscle. We put it under stress, which triggers the body to produce more. The trick is keeping that 'stress level' under the threshold of pain/injury. If your baseline is a higher 'level' of fit, you can get away with more stress (and fun!), with less repercussions! In fact, then they often just add to your strength and well-being overall, so bring it on!

I have a very specific workout routine/method that works for me. It took some time for me to get it where I wanted it for long-term. But that is part of the process. We are all different in what our ideal fitness level is, our ideal weight, our ideal routine and content, our ideal time of day, etc. We also all have different factors that come into play, when it comes to previous injuries/medical conditions/life situations. There are a lot of methods to lose weight or get fit. And, honestly, many of them work just fine. The part that makes them 'work' or not is often more about whether you can sustain it…and whether you can make it a habit and stick to it. The habit part is the difference-maker in most of these cases.

The trick, I think, is thinking more long-term. As long as you are moving TOWARDS your goal in a sustainable and healthy fashion, you ARE doing it. If you try to 'get there' before your mind AND body are on board, it can be a very frustrating and roller-coaster ride. You may even 'reach' your goal, but then 2 months later, realize you are drastically losing ground instead of maintaining what you worked so hard to achieve. Body break-down, unrealistic time requirements, or just plain fatigue can take you out of the game.

Think trajectory, not immediate attainment. Put your rewards along the way because you SHOULD be rewarding yourself, not abusing yourself. If you are on track or moving towards your goal, even if it is very gradual, that is worth celebrating. Be your own cheerleader. You deserve some praise. Change is challenging! But, it does not need to be a miserable process! Remember: step-wise, gradual, consistent. In fact, build in plateaus into your plan. I know, people tend to think of 'plateauing' as a negative thing when it comes to exercise/losing weight. Nope! Plateau so you SOLIDIFY your new baseline. Let it be your time to celebrate - it is your new, higher foundation. Make sure what you've built is sturdy and maintainable! Let your body have time to adjust to it and be non-reactive to it.

I debated whether to share any more details about my personal routine because: 1) Everyone is different and you have different underlying challenges and needs; 2) I am not here to tell you what's right for you, because I don't believe there is one 'right' for fitness/exercise. I believe there are a plethora of options! But, I do want to help any of you who are interested in what I have found to work for me. So, I will just include some details here. Keep in mind, I built this gradually and with many adaptations through other medical issues and past injuries. I also built this 'on top of' the basic habits from Chapter 5.

I wanted a balance of muscle strength and cardio fitness, that I felt would serve me best for whatever life throws at me. I also used the cardio portion to train my system to withstand more activity with less passing-out-ness (my own weird non-diagnosed medical condition mentioned earlier - it's been a challenge!). I learned personally just how important baseline-and-build could be. I also knew how important core/abdominal strength was for protection and optimal function for the rest of the body. I ALSO had many injuries from my past to take into consideration. All of that said, I set out to find my best workout routine for life moving forward.

Here is where my 5/7ths rule came into play. I gave/give myself 2 days off every week. But, overall, in an average week, I have a very specific routine the other 5 days of the week. I adapt as appropriate when it comes to travel, specific event plans, and other-people plans. I feel strongly about health/fitness, but I also feel strongly about fully enjoying what life has to offer. The reason it all works so well is the balance between the two. That is what is so wonderful about habits. If it is your overall 'normal,' then giving yourself leeway when it matters most to you is just part of the reward of taking care of yourself. Once the routine/habit is in place, you do not have to worry about temporary shifts/modifications/rest! You just get right back on routine afterwards (or you put your travel-routine version in the mix… or you bask in the 'break' altogether).

Ok. The simplest way to explain my routine is this: Monday, Wednesday, Friday are Abs + strengthening. This means I do a short (10-15 minutes) ab-specific routine, followed by a focus on essentially one half of the body for strengthening. So, Monday: Abs + upper body. Wednesday: Abs + lower body. Friday: Abs + combo of upper and lower and cardio. On Tuesday and Thursday: cardio (plus a 10 min gym-style bigger-muscle-group strengthening routine using machines). This may sound complicated, but it is pretty simple in terms of a balance of cardio (2-3 times per week) and strengthening (2-3 times per week). The thing to think about is making sure you are targeting the whole body, so you don't end up only working a few muscles over and over, creating strength/ weakness imbalances. You are going for whole-body fitness because this is a long-term program for yourself. Your whole self!

That is my 5-day/week routine. This does not mean you need to work out 5 days a week. You may find your ideal fitness level involves working out 2-3 days a week. The time you spend, the type of exercise, the activities you do outside of your baseline routine, and your life situation all weigh in. I found through the years that the key to a consistent healthy fitness level is more about establishing the habit of exercise 'for general health' than it is about the exact routine. I have also been through unexpected life changes, medical conditions, injuries, etc. that have tested and challenged it. But, the reason I was able to overcome all of these things and not spiral towards overall decline was the reminder to myself to use what I DID have functioning throughout all the challenges. I kept the habit, even if I had to make some major adaptations to the content. Use what you have. I had very little use of one side of my upper body for an extended period of time. I had a lot of pain. I had other health issues kicking in hard. I had emotional stress. I lived alone. I also knew I had it really good compared to a lot of people out there that have no or little use of their limbs.

Early in my physical therapy career, I worked with a patient who had been severely burned (electrocuted) all over his body. He lost most of all 4 limbs. He was a torso. And he was one of the most amazing people I will ever meet. I think of him every time I think I have it rough. He made the most of every day and he worked hard every day to improve his condition, however he could. He used what he had. He strengthened what he had. And he was amazing. And, he was happy. I learned so many things from working with him that I keep with me today.

I thought of all that I learned from him while I worked on getting myself back to 'baseline.' I used all parts of me that were usable. I was grateful for what I did have, and I made sure to take care of the rest of me so it could help take care of my less-than-ideal 'broken' parts. And, I knew my goal. I knew it was going to be slower than I wanted, harder than I wanted, and that there would be obstacles. But, I knew I just had to re-calculate. Move forward. Keep whatever pieces of my 'routine' that I could and modify as needed. I walked every day, even though at first I could only manage 5 minutes. But, I could walk. So, I did. Eventually, I got back to 30 minutes/day. Eventually (years) I got back to my baseline workout. Not everyone is that lucky. Some life-happenings mean you can no longer do what you used to do. But, you can do what you can. And you can be happy doing it. Life is too short not to.

When I was re-calculating… I made a plan, I got my mind and body on board, and I know I would be in a much different state today if I had not. Besides, we are all an accumulation of all our injuries, our experiences, and our victories. Some things can't be fixed or corrected, and some goals have to be re-gained to sustain (or re-calibrated to achieve). As long as you are moving towards the positive, you are winning out over the spiraling negative. As long as your habits are engineered to propel you forward, you ARE on track.

Whatever goal you pick, if it's an ideal weight goal or a fitness-specific goal, you can think of the 'step-wise and plateau' part as your building blocks. First, pick a very specific and realistic starting point, based on your current baseline 'normal.' For instance, maybe pick a 30-minute routine to do 2 times per week to start. Make sure it is not at the expense of your 10 daily habits. You are building. Do your new routine consistently for 3 weeks. Don't be too gung-ho about increasing it quickly. Just get the body-handles-it-well-and-so-does-your-schedule thing going. Figure out what time of day works best, the logistics of where/space you are going to use, prime up your excuse-busting strength, etc.

Think of it this way. Once you have started the habit (30 min, 2x/week), you can look forward to the thought that after 3 weeks of doing this consistently, the initial habit-starting-to-stick part will be on your side! As you build and continue the routine, you can look forward to the 3-month mark as a more solidified and fortified habit!

Habit change and physical body (and brain) changes go together when it comes to fitness goals. I would think of it as: First 3 weeks = habit starting to 'stick'… First 3 months = habit starting to 'stay.' Even after 3 months, you can still get 'out of the habit' obviously, BUT it is more ingrained and easier to get 'back IN the habit.' The first 3 weeks, you are getting over the initial habit-starting hump. So, at 3 weeks you should definitely celebrate! You did the extra-hard part! As you are moving towards the 3 months, know that more and more physical changes are happening to assist you (both brain and body). Add to this the understanding that if you start strengthening a particular muscle, the first 3-4 weeks you are just improving the brain-to-muscle pathway part of strengthening (this is a big part of the process). Your body can only produce new muscle, as in creating more muscle mass, so quickly. That part becomes part of the deal after 3-4 weeks. So, consider the first month your habit-strengthening phase.

After 3-4 weeks, you will be making physical changes to the muscle as well. By 3 months, you will have BOTH brain and body physical changes on your side. More solidified habit + more muscle mass = EXTRA celebration!! By the way, you can 'feel' stronger in a muscle well before 3 weeks. Just realize the body can only naturally produce more muscle mass so fast. The initial few weeks are increasing the neural pathway 'strength,' so to speak. So, coordination/signals to the muscle are improving first. This can also feel like increased strength, because, well, it is all part of the process. So, you can certainly feel stronger even before your body has had the chance to build the muscle itself. Ok, good! So, landmark celebrations at 3 weeks and 3 months. Be sure to celebrate/reward yourself for everything in between, of course. Every single day/week that you follow-through is a congratulatory day/week in my opinion!

Ok!! This is where we combine everything we've talked about so far. Drink some water, if you have not since you started this book please. I am doing the same. Yes, thank you! Get up and dance around. Yep, same. Readjust the pillow behind your back. Nope. I am sitting up straight while typing on my balcony, but thank you again. Breathe in and out 5 deep breaths. That felt good. Ok. We are ready.

You know your What and Why. You've gotten your brain behind you/working for you. You are planning a step-wise, gradual workout program that is realistic and sustainable. You are thinking of all the things/excuses that may try to thwart your plan. You are getting all of these excuses out of the equation before they even show up. You are setting yourself up to be reliable to yourself, not to let yourself down. You know your Why is your health and well-being, so you are prioritizing it like your health and well-being depends on it… um, it does. If you are not healthy, fit, and strong (in whatever ways your body allows), then everything else gets harder to maintain as well. You are reminding yourself you only have one body. One. You want to help it run as efficiently as possible for all the things it gets to do (and has to overcome). You know it's all fun and games until it breaks down on you due to neglect. Ok, you're ready.

Whatever routine you decide on, you want to incorporate your new body-position habits as best as you can:

1) **Proper 'set' position (back straight, shoulders slightly back, chin slightly tucked)**
2) **TA activation (lower abs engage!)**
3) **No locked knees or hip drop**

Oh! And, please don't forget to breathe (don't hold your breath during reps or exercise in general… or in life… in general). And hydrate! And stretch. Excellent.

If you are doing reps of weights sitting or standing, just try to incorporate the 'set' position as much as you can, given the action you are doing. You are integrating the 'set' position and Ab activation to protect yourself, as well as to stabilize yourself for the best alignment/form you can attain while stressing (in the safe and pain-free way) the muscles you are trying to strengthen.

If you are doing reps, let's say on a weight machine of some kind in the gym, be mindful of your start and end position for each rep. It should be in a range of motion that does not stress the joints themselves. This is where the 'set' position can be very helpful for guidance. The shoulder position may seem tricky (don't do anything bizarre just to try to keep your shoulders slightly back), but just remember you are trying to keep your joints/muscles in good posture overall. Your shoulders are ball-joints. This means they can go in a lot of different directions within the joint. You are trying to keep the 'ball' of the joint in the center of its little safe home. If your shoulders creep forward from the center, you are now allowing the bone to move towards tendons and other tissues. This means that you could be fraying (due to friction) muscle/tendon that can lead to shoulder strain/tearing. So, 'center' your shoulders by being mindful of avoiding 'forward shoulders.' Much like 'setting' your abs, you are just putting yourself in the most protected scenario, and then adding the exercise to it.

It is also good to keep in mind that the slower you move through a rep, the harder it is for the muscle you are targeting. This is good for strengthening! So, don't speed through! For one, it is a more effective way to strengthen. And two, it is more likely you are actually accurately targeting the one muscle you are intentionally trying to work. Speed can cause other muscle groups to kick in to try to help out. This is a version of compensation. If you slow down a bit, to be sure you can keep a good body position AND target the right muscle, you will be much more effective and efficient in your strengthening routine.

By the way, you certainly don't need a gym to have a good

exercise routine. I just use those examples for ease of description. You can target and strengthen any muscle, just by using a combination of body weight (floor-type) exercise, dumbbells, and/or exercise bands/tubing. Many people (like me) just find it's easier to use the gym for cardio (keeping things low-impact like bike and elliptical) and for targeting certain bigger muscle groups like lat pull-downs and rows for example. That said, that is just what works best for me as my 'normal' routine. I have back-up routines for when I am traveling, etc., where a gym is not an easy option. If I did not have a gym nearby, I would just create a non-gym plan. I have traveled for months at a time internationally and domestically and just switch to a non-gym version. See… contingency planning… quite helpful!

Let's talk a bit about Abs and cardio together! To use me as an example, I use the elliptical machine (in place of running) to get some good (low impact) cardio work. While I am elliptical-ing, I just do intermittent reps of lower ab contraction. Well, I should back up. I have done it long enough that I now notice when I am NOT using my lower abs and then kick them in. But, this takes some time. So, technically, I have them engaged (intentionally, but rarely have to think about it) most of the time while doing standing cardio. But, unless you have trained them over time already, you want to gradually add them into your routine just like you are with walking.

Start small. Try the same routine as with walking in that maybe you just do a 5 sec on/5 sec off for 1-2 minutes at the beginning and the end of your cardio session. Get used to that first. Then you can gradually increase the frequency as your body (and you, mentally) tolerate! You don't want to freak out your back (or your mind) by all of a sudden trying to use your abs for long periods of time when you are not used to it. The great news is that the more you start to integrate lower abs into the rest of your program, the stronger they get along the way… and no extra time required! So, in sum, you will be strengthening your abs and your postural muscles along with the rest of your workout targets. Whehoo!

Life is about balance. Make sure whatever goal/s you set for yourself line up with your true desires/beliefs. Make sure they line up with True You. Setting goals that rely on (or are underneath-it-all, FOR) others are a different ball game. I don't mean you shouldn't do things for others in your life, I am just talking about your very personal goals. No matter who is (or isn't) in your life does not factor in here. I know, that sounds insensitive (or something), but this is ALL. ABOUT. YOU. People can come in and out of your life for many different reasons. This can be awesome or less-than-awesome, but these goals are things that you are creating for YOU. Be selfish, in the best way possible. You should be. Taking care of yourself allows you to be your best possible healthy self. This sets you up to be your best self in whatever else you do and in whatever relationships you have with others on this (amazing and mysterious) planet!

Ok, people! It's time to LAUNCH. You have a goal, you have a plan, your thoughts/brain support you, your body has a daily habit foundation to support you… so, it's official Go-Time! All you need is the DECISION part. You need belief + action to carry this through.

The official moment you decide, you need to be fully 'in.' So… let's do it. It's happening. This is a great moment. You should feel it. Know it. Celebrate it. The moment you truly decide, consider it DONE. If you have done the prep work, it IS done. It is just you in the future. Which is coming. So, then, it's done!

It is liberating in the same way as getting out of decision debt! Once you make a decision (for real), you are now officially free of the indecision. Get behind yourself 100%. Make. It. Happen. Be your own best friend. Be reliable. And (hopefully) be excited! You are choosing to do something important for yourself. The 'work' will be worth it, if you regard yourself as a priority in your own life and follow through. Set a date. LAUNCH!!

Tips:

1. **Make a REAL decision and have a REAL plan**
2. **Know your What and Why**
3. **Brain on Board (thoughts match goal)**
4. **Body on Board (realistic starting point given current body baseline)**
5. **Step-wise, gradual, and consistent (plateaus are good!)**
6. **Stay under threshold of pain/inflammation**
7. **Contingency plans/excuse-busters already in place**

Oh and ...

8. **Build in rewards/freedom!**

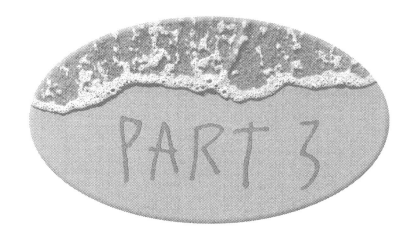

The Bucket List:
Get After It

CHAPTER 7

X factor = Happiness Factor

Question for you. I'm just curious. Do you have a bucket list? Just on the off chance you don't know what this is, I will explain. A bucket list is a list of things you REALLY want to do before you die, or as the saying goes, before you 'kick the bucket.'

I don't ever remember NOT having a bucket list. Maybe that is weird. I don't know; that is why I am extra curious to know if you even have one now. I don't like to assume, so I am going to presume instead. I am going to presume that you do because most everyone I know does have some version of a bucket list. But, maybe the better question is... are you actively pursuing it? Now, let me just say, no pressure... unless you truly want to do these things (or that one thing). Ha. So, no pressure from me, only a friendly reminder of the whole life-is-short thing. As Jack Kornfield says in *Buddha's Little Instruction Book*, 'The trouble is that you think you have time.' After working for so many years with patients who all of a sudden had life-changing injuries or conditions, I was constantly reminded of this. And for me, for whatever reason, it's always been at the forefront of my mind (as long as I can remember) and not the back burner. I don't know if this is good or bad, it is just me.

The thing is, so many people have all the reasons/excuses why they are not actively moving towards their list. And I get it 100%. I had a lot of reasons and excuses not to as well. But, since life (as we know it) is finite and an undetermined length, well, that changes the equation. At least in my mind it does. My hope for all of you is that you can use this part of the book to inspire you... remind you... motivate you... excite you... towards actually ACTING on these things that you want to do!

I know I am possibly a somewhat extreme case of early

bucket-listing, which also turned into 'early' acting on it. I knew very young that I did not want to wait for retirement or the perfect time or any of the things that lead to inaction, when it came to taking advantage of all that life and this planet had to offer. And, I can say that every single thing that I set out to do, or experience, was more than worth whatever work or risk or excuse-busting it took to make it happen. In short, no regrets. Ever. I think that is the thing about your bucket list. You KNOW you want to do it, it's not a maybe. You are genuinely deep-down motivated to do whatever it is, so regrets are not even in the mix.

This does not mean everything has been smooth sailing. Nope! But, completely and amazingly worth it. Every time. By the way, everyone's list is different, but the common denominator is that for YOU (the list-maker)… it is kick-ass! If it is the top of the list of things you want to do before you die, then by default, it is amazing! And the great thing is there can be no judgement. Let me rephrase that... who cares what anyone else thinks about your list - it is YOUR list. It could be traveling to a far-off country, or it could be underwater basket weaving. It could be skydiving, or it could be planting a succulent garden. It could be seeing U2 play live in Dublin, or it could be learning to play the drums. Um, yes, some of these examples may apply to me. But, my point is it could be anything. And it is all awesome, if it is your true Happy-List.

I think of bucket lists as 2 categories:

1) **Single - event (although some got repeated in my case)**
2) **Daily - life.**

For instance, one of my single-event items was seeing World Cup soccer in Brazil. Granted, I combined it with a 2.5-month South American solo travel adventure (2 items in 1)! For me, seeing South America AND seeing World Cup matches in Brazil was a must-do. I had to put a job on the line, a relationship on the line, save for years etc., but it was 100% worth every bit. The day the World Cup host nation was announced, I made the decision to go. That gave me 8 years to save. And I did. One year later, I had another top item come into play when the US Women's World Cup team made it to the finals. Another must-do for me! That one wasn't the kind of thing I could plan for, but I knew when it happened, I would find a way to go. These both fell under Category #1.

Another Category #1 for me was seeing U2 play Dublin. The first time I did this (yes, this one may have gotten repeated... um, multiple times in the years to follow), I combined it with an extended Ireland trip. Ireland was a place I had wanted to go as far back as I can remember. In fact, going to Ireland was my first bucket list item (I believe starting at age 3). I know, weird! Since then, I have been many times and I consider it one of my top happy-places.

Category #1 also has included things like skydiving, paragliding, hot air ballooning, parasailing, scuba diving the great barrier reef, etc. It's funny, you would think bungee jumping might be on there if I have a thrill-seeking thing going on, but NOT AT ALL. I have zero desire to do that. Jumping out of planes, running off of mountains, watching sharks swim by... were all great, but jumping with a rope attached to my limb... apparently not my thing! Oh! Now, this one I have to mention because it was one of the most amazing things (and probably not on most people's radar)... swimming with manatees. Manatees have been my favorite animal since I was a kid. I think something about their friendly nature, they have no enemies, and they are playful creatures... I can't get enough of them. Swimming with them in their natural environment and seeing just how playful they really are, makes my heart so happy just remembering it. One of them swam underneath my dad's treading-water feet and slowly lifted him up out of the water! Adorable creatures and so amazing to experience.

Just as important (for me) as these big single-event type experiences are/were, I get just as excited about the daily-life bucket list things in my life. Learning to play guitar and learning to play the drums are just as fulfilling as the single-event things. The daily-life items bring joy into daily life, whereas the single-event items bring joy in the moment (and through their memories). For me, being able to walk to the beach, play the drums, and go hiking all bring me joy that I want in my everyday life. So, I made that a reality.

Enough about me. I want to delve into YOUR life a bit. Let's go back to Chapter 1 for a minute. Remember the 2 lists you made: 1) 3 things you enjoyed as a kid 2) 3 things you love to do today. Look at both lists and consider what MOST excites you (or calms you). In short, which ones give you the most joy/happiness if you could have them as part of your daily life. This could be daily or weekly or monthly overall, but we will call it 'daily life' for ease. If there are any from your kid-list that you want back in your today-life, add it to the today list. Make this your official Daily-Life Bucket List.

Let's take just a moment for a preview of the extra fun part as well. Start contemplating your Single-event Bucket List, too. As we are going along in the remaining chapters, update/dream/ contemplate this list so that by the time we get to Chapter 9, you are ready for the crazy-good stuff!

Ok, now, let's think about how we can make your Daily-Life Bucket List come to life! Just like brain habits and body habits, we can use the same process to create your Bucket List Habits! You see, even the things you truly enjoy and WANT to do often get put on the back burner due to all the things you feel you HAVE to do first. We even procrastinate doing the things we truly want to do, even if we DO have the time. But let's look at the former. I agree to some extent, there are things you really have to do. We all know how that feels. And we are all different in how we prioritize, depending on our life situations. BUT, if you never prioritize your happy-list, then you do all the HAVE-TOs which leave out... you. I also agree that, just as I have structured this book in a certain order, brain and body health ARE things you should prioritize in your everyday life first. So, you might wonder (or exclaim), 'There is not enough time in a day, woman!' Yep. I know that thought, too. Let's rewind. We want our thoughts supporting us, not working against us. Part I coming at you hard again! It is relentless, I know. But it works. It just does.

You do have time. It may not seem like it at first. You just have to decide you do. I hear you, 'sure, sure, easy for you to say all chillin' by the beach writing and drumming while I am here taking care of 5 kids and working full time and walking uphill both ways...' Well, true (ish) for me and maybe that is your situation (that's rough), but think of the same process as adding the 5 minutes in your day for brain-not-on-fire. Think about it as just 5 minutes of you-time.

If that is truly all you can spare in your current situation, then there you go.

I live in a one-room... um, not brand new...studio apartment. Most of my furniture and belongings (from a bigger apartment in Seattle) lived on my balcony for a month before I could figure out what made the cut to fit inside. Luckily it did not rain a single day (although it did rain the day after I got everything inside that I was going to keep!) while I was in transition. I have no couch, but I have 2 drum kits. It's true. My point is, you make room (and time) for what matters to you most. The WHAT is not right or wrong, it is whatever is right for you, given the current situation. But there are sacrifices, of course. So, if you need to purge some not-so-crucially-important-to-you activities (cough, mindless Instafacing, just a possibility) to make some room/time for 5-10 minutes of learning a chord on guitar or tending to your succulents or reading about how to basket-weave underwater, or whatever floats your boat/brings you joy... well, then 5 minutes it is! Once you have the new habit of 5 minutes devoted to your new hobby/joy-time in your day, I think you will miraculously find even more time. Or, you will find ways to purge something else. Or you will rearrange your schedule slightly (or massively) to accommodate something important, for more joy moments in your life.

The habit itself is the key. You could even just sit with your succulents for 5 minutes, if they bring you joy. You could learn a new funk beat on drums. You could use that 5 minutes to plan how to create that 5 minutes (or more)! Some days I can play 30 minutes on drums and it is glorious! Some days I may only get 5 minutes. But, guess what, it is STILL glorious.

To me, life is really a bunch of wonderfully special moments, interspersed with the not-so-wonderful. The more joy-moments you create for yourself, the more you can appreciate every single day. No matter who is in your life, and no matter what you are going through. Even if you are going through truly terrible things (it's going to happen), you can use your happy-habits to interrupt and counter the rough stuff as much as possible. In the end, it is about enjoying what life we do have and making the most of it. Sometimes the little things, the 5-minute things, are actually gigantic things when it comes to happiness. They are beautiful reminders of the life-is-short-so-do-what-you-love-while-you-can thing. It's a thing.

Ok, so now that you have taken Daily-Life Bucket List inventory, let's narrow it down to your top 3. These are your top 3 things you want to incorporate in/back into your life. Make sure they are truly yours, not someone else's. I know that sounds weird but dig deep here. These are your top 3 activities you enjoy the most. By the way, bucket list things for daily life may involve doing LESS, not more. I say this because for many of us, what would bring more joy is actually taking time to enjoy something by doing less. If that makes any sense.

For me, being at the beach is relaxing and calming. I call it my wave-sound therapy. It is one of my favorite things 'to do.' Drumming is quite different. It uses a completely different part of my brain to make 4 limbs do 4 separate things, at once. It is addictive in that it feels impossible until... it's not. And when it clicks, it is one of the best feelings! I never get bored and I always want more. Hiking is calming and active all at the same time. These are my top 3 at the moment, and they all have very different effects on me. But, all 3 of them bring me great joy. Of course, there are many other things as well, but I specify these, so you know what I mean when I suggest narrowing to your top 3.

The possibilities are endless and there are no right or wrong choices. It could be gardening, reading, a sport, learning or playing an instrument, or doing a hobby of any kind. If the 5-min/day plan doesn't work or is not suitable for a particular starting point (let's say your #1 is adding basketball back in as we discussed as an earlier example), then think more of a 30 min/week idea. Whatever gets it in your life-routine. We are just thinking of the habit-formation part right now. You are game-planning, considering what you may need to purge, establishing your list.

Daily-Life Bucket List Top 3:

#1. _____

#2. _____

#3. _____

It's a weird concept to have to MAKE a habit of something you already know you WANT to do, but it's part of helping yourself help yourself. Once you get the habit going (we will discuss more next chapter), you will realize how much it truly adds to your life and you will devise ways to keep it/include it/bolster it! It's getting the activation energy to START that holds so many people back from doing things they DO want to do. If you've ever heard Mel Robbins speak (I love her), you know about the insanely-simple-yet-effective

5-4-3-2-1 rule. It's ridiculous that it works, but it has worked for me over and over. It is just getting your brain working FOR you in all its simplicity/complexity!

If you are not familiar with Mel's use of the 5-4-3-2-1 rule, I will explain. In sum, you can help your brain help you get started (in the moment) by just simply counting down from 5 and then ACTION. She describes it wonderfully in her TED talks, etc., but that is the gist. She used it to get herself out of bed (literally), to get her life going in a positive direction, and ultimately to change her life completely. I use it, too. Thank you, Mel! It is also fascinating on the brain side because of the way our brain gives us about 5 seconds to act on a thought, before all the self-doubt or procrastination or reasons NOT to act kick in to stop you.

She explains all of these things more thoroughly, but I throw it in here because ACTION is what you need to get started. Counting down from 5 in a 5-4-3-2-1-GO scenario helps make it happen in the moment. Efficient AND effective - right up my alley! Anything that helps interrupt your procrastination-brain (or fear or self-doubt or anything else stopping you from taking a step, taking action, no matter how small) and to overcome inaction, is worth knowing about when it comes to creating new habits.

I like to think of starting something in terms of physics. I love physics when applied (in my weird way) to simple daily-life activities. For instance, I think of the Law of Inertia (Newton's First Law of Motion) anytime I am starting a new habit. This law states that 'an object at rest remains at rest, or if in motion, remains in motion at a constant velocity unless acted on by a new external force.' Now, in purely physics terms, this force could be friction, air resistance, gravity, etc. But for us, think of it in terms of current habits (already in motion), or new habits not-yet-begun (inaction, at rest).

We need to create the net external force to change the trajectory, velocity, or its static vs active state. Habits, once they 'stick' help provide the remain-in-motion part! We just need the activation energy part (the net external force part)!

In chemistry, activation energy is defined as the minimum energy required to start a reaction. An easy example would be lighting a match. When you strike the match, the energy/friction you created is what initiated the combustion reaction. Fire! So, light a fire under your own ass, so to speak (please note the so-to-speak part)! Count it down. Whatever gets you to produce your own activation energy, use it.

I want to go a little further into the digging-deep part of all this bucket listing. You can use some of the tools from Part I to really get into what you genuinely want/enjoy out of life. It sounds strange, but remember when I mentioned the idea of posing a question to yourself before you go to sleep? You simply pose the question mentally (I suppose you could do it audibly if you want) and then let it go to your subconscious for the night. For me, I may ask for clarity on some particular challenge or decision in my life. I then picture that question making its way to the deeper part of my brain to hang out for the night. I picture the question tucking itself in there for the rest of the night. I do this because it helps 'release' it from my conscious brain so that I am not actively thinking about it anymore while I am trying to go to sleep. I want my brain on sleepy-mode, not on figure-this-out mode.

When you first wake, use the groggy time to notice your

thoughts, as discussed. You may not have a massive light bulb moment, but you may get some insight. I've had all versions of both, as well as just 'huh' moments with no particular insight. But then, often later, the 'huh' moments are elevated to 'HUH!" moments. The same type of things have happened after 5-minute meditations. Just sayin', it's worth a go!

You may not need these tools to figure out what you truly want out of life, but you may get little nuggets that add to or support what you already know. Some people could make their list easily (and already have) and know it comes from somewhere deep inside of them. For others, this is difficult to do with clarity. I found that when you truly give yourself a 'stop and assess' chance, you can connect to your deeper self, your intuition, and your genuine happy-life factors. They are sometimes hiding underneath a LOT of … life-so-far-ness and old repeated thought patterns about yourself that no longer (or never did) actually serve you. Or, you may realize just how many things that you currently do are not serving you at all, just others. You may find that what you thought made you happy really just made others happy/more comfortable.

Of course, I do know and feel that making others happy can be a great ADDITION to your happiness. As long as you pay attention to the difference, and make sure you are paying attention to your own needs, that just becomes an extra plus. If you are neglecting your own needs amidst all the taking-care-of-others' needs, things can get murky (and in the long-run, just plain muddy). If you take some time to tune in to YOU, you will discover the stand-alone happy factors in all of this. If you think eliminating decision debt is liberating, hold onto your scotch and drum sticks people! Or, tea and reading glasses. Whatever you have on you. The moment you know FOR SURE what you want, it is KABLAM-level liberating! You will know when you hit KABLAM-level. I have found it takes a few things to get there. It takes an earnest look at yourself including:

1) **Being vulnerable and honest with yourself**
2) **Not judging yourself**
3) **Eliminating noise pollution (both internal and external)**
4) **Being you, using your personal internal compass (use it, it's in there!)**

CHAPTER 8

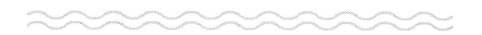

Habits to Happiness

In the Introduction of this book, I gave some insight into my somewhat extreme personal 're-set' of my life when I entered my 40s. For me, it became very clear I needed major changes. What wasn't so clear at first was what exactly those changes would look like. I knew I needed a job change. I knew I needed a location change. I also knew I wasn't going to get full clarity on these things immediately. I knew I was going to need to fully tune into my internal compass in a big way and allow myself to discover it as a process. I also knew I needed to do all the things I listed at the end of Chapter 7.

I knew that I didn't have the finances to keep an apartment while figuring it all out, including where my new home would be. I knew I needed clarity, and I needed to take care of my mind and body along the way. In sum, I had to let go of all my comfort/security zones to allow myself to dig extra deep and find my way.

Given all of this, I put my belongings in storage and in space created for me by two very loving friends (thank you Kari and Lori!). By the way, these two also gave me recovery space in their homes at some very challenging moments in the process. True friends can be life-savers… if you let them. I have a (understatement) hard time accepting help and these two, along with my dad, made sure I had it despite my strong tendencies to decline it!

While I was getting off sleep aids and in a VERY reduced mental state, my dad gave me what was probably the only place I could have managed to get through it (my old bedroom and his gentle presence in the house with me). I don't remember much of this time period. When I say I didn't sleep for a while, that is a massive understatement. Thinking back on it, I truly don't know how I survived those months. That may sound dramatic, but it is indescribable, that period of time in my life. However, I knew, somehow, it was absolutely necessary, and I had to get through it and to the 'other side.' I needed to train my body to learn how to sleep again. And I needed that in order to get clarity on my life. However long it took.

I officially hit the re-set button HARD on my life. The full realization it needed to happen was in my 41st year. That is when I put my stuff in storage, left my job, left Seattle, and left the country. When I returned to the US, the real work began. I was ready, I just wasn't sure what it would all entail, where I would end up, or how much I would go through to get to today. I am now 43. It was quite a journey, to say the least! There were so many practical-me reasons not to do what I did, when it comes to finances/security/comfort zones. And, it took everything I had to make sure those things did not stop me from finding my way.

I packed my car in Seattle and headed on an internal-compass journey to find 'my place.' That journey itself could be a book of its own, but the end result was unmistakable and unquestionable. It is hard to describe what it took to suspend/block all the 'input' coming at me that was based on… logic… practicality…pragmatism. It was a battle between those parts of me and my intuition. I created a space in myself that would only listen to my gut/intuition. It was not easy. I made the decision, before I left Seattle, to go on a search that had no determined destination (other than that all my senses said to start with CA). No small place! I also made the decision that if I got to a place that 'grabbed' me aggressively and immediately upon arrival, I would know that was the place.

It happened exactly that way. When I got to Carlsbad, CA, my insides flipped out in a way I cannot describe. It was shocking and intense. And unmistakable. The weirdest thing. From that moment, I knew this was the place I was going to recover and start my new chapter in life. Little did I know, it would also involve these 9 chapters!

I do realize that a drastic change like this and everything that went with it along the way (so many health issues and challenges), is not necessarily something any of you will experience. But, some of you may. Every one of us is different, our life circumstances are different, our needs and desires are different, our priorities are different. But, I think, deep down we all have the same thing inside of us - the pursuit of happiness. How we choose to pursue it, what we are dealt in life as obstacles, and what creates happiness for each of us is what makes things interesting! And unique. And totally worth the pursuit.

My feelings on happiness are vast. And I know you can be happy no matter what your situation, because it is inside. However, if there are things you CAN change, things you CAN pursue, that you know deep down would significantly add to your daily happiness, well, hell, I am all for pursuing it!

We come up with all kinds of reasons to hold ourselves back. Most of them are based on fear and/or self-doubt. I have those things, too (yep, it's true!), I just choose to act anyway. I had to make the decision to push through them head-on. I heard Mel Robbins say (told you I love her!), 'self-doubt is a habit and worry is a habit.' It's so true. She also said, 'If you have a problem that can be solved with action, then you don't have a problem.' Also, so true! One more… 'confidence is the decision to try and self-doubt is the decision NOT to try.' Just sayin'… I can relate to her thoughts so intensely because I came to these same conclusions in my personal journey. All of these things are worth thinking about as you contemplate your own happy-factors in life!

What you want and what you are naturally good at don't always go together. I say this because so many people talk about your 'purpose' and your 'gift' and how you should share it with the world. I agree 100%. Unless that thing you are so good at is not actually what makes you happy. If it doesn't feed your soul, then I think it is worth considering putting your energy into things that do.

For some people, what they want and what they are good at go together fantastically! I think that is awesome! All I am saying is that sometimes, I think we stick to a particular path because it is based on what we think we are good at and that must mean it is what we are supposed to be doing. And maybe that is true for you, and they match. I think it is worth taking a look at whether they match, or if it is just another reason to avoid change/stay in your comfort zone. Whatever your particular situation, just consider ways you can put more energy into the things you really are passionate about. Even if right now it's only in 5-minute bursts!

The hard part in all of this is the change itself, even if it's a great change. This applies to even the small things, like finding 5 minutes to do something you thoroughly enjoy. Adding a new happy-factor habit into your day is a change in your schedule or routine. As goofy as it sounds, this can be a really big deal! At the very least, you can start working on adding these small things into your life now. Then you can consider bigger changes that take some planning along the way. I do understand that most of you won't choose to do it all in one big mid-life crisis kind of way the way I did. But, hey, if you do, welcome to the massive-change-in-your-forties club!

Speaking of clubs! I am currently designing bucket list club retreats in CA wine country for women in their 40s, tackling and applying the concepts in this book WHILE enjoying life in the process! Some of you maybe even fall into an even more specific bucket list club category of women in your 40s who are marriage-free and kid-free. For those of you who can relate to this, I want you to know you are not alone! You may feel like you are going life alone (and in many ways you are), but you are certainly not alone in that there are MANY of us in this particular category right now! We do exist! And (I might be a little biased here), we tend to be quite unique people if you ask me! All those reasons feed into why I am also creating small-group retreats specifically for you.

Making changes, big and small when it comes to mind/body/life can be hard to do, even if you get the 'how-to' part. Sometimes, being able to relate to others in the same chapter in life and in similar circumstances can be just what you need to create the spark (activation energy!) to fully take charge of your life and happiness! If what I know from my background and what I have experienced in my life can help guide, inspire, and motivate you in going after your health and bucket list goals... (AND, do it in a relaxing environment)... well, that's MY goal. A lot of things happen (good and bad) in this particular time in our lives that actually make it the PERFECT time to re-set and re-boot!

So, let's re-set! You hopefully have your top 3 things you want in your daily life listed and anxiously waiting for you. Think of these Daily-Life Bucket List items much like your baseline health habits you've already created. These daily-life happy-factors need as much attention as your mind and body do, in order to make them a reality. So, make sure to use the same process (and patience) with yourself. These become your Happy-Factor Foundation! They just need some 'stick' (3 weeks) and 'stay' (3 months) habit-love from you!

Remember the baseline and build concept? Start small. 5 minutes/day. Or 5 min/day, 5 days/week. Or 5 min/day, 3 days/week. Or, if the activity is better suited per week, then 30 min/week. You choose. You will know what makes sense for the particular activity. Start with one. Give it a chance to enter your routine. Tweak, adapt, purge, excuse-bust. Don't overwhelm yourself. Purge what you need to. Let the other 2 happy factors be on deck (or hang out on your balcony) until you make room for them, too. And remember, sometimes it is all about LESS, not MORE. Your stress level should REDUCE adding these into your life, not increase! You are in the purge-and-replace game! Maybe pick a current not-so-awesome habit to purge and replace it with your new definitely-awesome happy-factor habit. This is even better, because you can use the cue that normally drives you to do a not-awesome habit and just replace the action in the middle (happy-factor habit). In the habit-formation world, this tends to be the most effective way to create a 'new' habit/change a bad habit. And bonus! Out with the bad, in with the good!

For some people, they discover that some of the purging process includes reducing time spent with certain people in your life as well. I don't mean drop all your great friends, no! I just mean, sometimes you realize there are people you put energy towards that are not actually a positive part of your life. And some are straight-up negative in terms of your well-being. Time is precious. I would just say consider ALL the aspects of how you currently use your time. That way, you can use this as a more complete re-set while you are working on finding ways to make your life better for you in the grand scheme.

You might also want to consider using this time to evaluate how you spend your money. I did a complete OVERHAUL given my circumstances, in order to make all these changes happen. If you haven't done a thorough evaluation in this area of your life recently, this the perfect time to do it. You may find you can purge certain things that are just on 'autopilot spend' that you realize are nowhere near necessary. This can help open things up to put your time/money/energy into new arenas that maybe serve to help you, your well-being, and your future adventures in life!

It is all about the choices you make. You are in control of your own happiness and how you go about creating it/building upon it. I hate to say it, but so often it is a person (or people) that hold so many people back. You may not even realize it. This is where self-doubt and fear can enter the scene bigtime! This is all tricky territory, I know. But, deep down you will know if change is needed. The question is whether you listen to it. Fear and self-doubt will be there lurking of course, but they don't have to win. You get to decide who wins. It is your life. You are the only one who truly knows what is best for you. You just have to be brave enough to go after what is on the other side of fear. If it is right, deep down, then it is right. And yes, it can be full-on scary and messy and uncomfortable. In fact, these often are the signs that you are on the right track! In my experience, it has been well worth the scary and the messy and the uncomfortable (many times over in my life, not just in my 40s), to get to a place that is based on truth, not fear.

Whew. That got deep. Ok, let's integrate! You have your 10 daily health habits going, you have your 5-min brain-NOT-on-fire habit going, you have your weekly (starter) workout habit going, and now you have your first happy-factor daily-life bucket list habit going. Ok, if you are just reading for now, and none of these have happened yet, I still love you! But I hope you are at least in the process and are creating the space for them.

Ok, so, here is where everything so far gets to play together! Let's say your new happy-factor habit is a sitting activity. If it is playing an instrument, or painting, or reading, or gardening, or so many other possibilities… then we want to apply everything we learned in Part II. When I started playing drums every day, I 'installed' the habit of sitting upright with good posture right from the start. If you train yourself early, with a new activity, it's just part of the new habit. New activity means it is new for your mind AND your body. These are great things! Learning new things is good for the brain, we just want to be sure it is also as good as possible for the body in the process.

If you train yourself in the early stages of the new activity, it is much easier than adding in good posture/body mechanics later. It also reduces the chances that the new activity/hobby turns into a sad-face hobby for your body! Even 5 minutes per day adds up, when it comes to what your body is doing/what it is used to doing.

If your new hobby is a sport-type activity, integrating what you know about the body and muscle changes can be a big deal as well. Let's say you are now playing 30 min -1 hour of a new sport 1x/week. Sounds excellent! Just keep in mind that sometimes the body (yep, we are in our 40s, it happens), will unexpectedly flip out on you! I know, you didn't have a problem playing 10 sports at once when you were younger. I know. But see, the body doesn't always react the way you expect when you add up all the years of what you have done and well, all the years. It may feel just fine while you are playing and so you play longer than you planned, and you are a happy-camper sportsing your heart out. And then, BLAM. Or, and then, the next day, BLAM. Or, some version of BLAM a couple weeks later. Sometimes a new activity can set off an inflammatory response or muscle spasms or old-injury alignment issues that we don't expect from a single seemingly harmless activity.

So, let's try to prevent this from happening to you. A couple of suggestions here. 1) Consider all the prevention strategies discussed in Part II. 2) Consider your posture/body mechanics/ repetitive movement involved in the new sport/activity and incorporate these things proactively. This includes counter-stretching, counter-strengthening, and counter-movements. 3) Be GRADUAL in your approach and let your body catch up to the new routine! You are basically just making sure you are gradually increasing the activity at a rate under the threshold of pain/inflammation. 4) Understand your body may not give you OBVIOUS warning, so you should be thinking consistency (and build in plateauing) while you are starting/progressing a sport, even if you feel fine doing it.

I know it sounds like I am taking the fun out of playing a sport, but believe me, I am just making sure you get to CONTINUE the fun of the sport itself! It can be a little annoying to think about all of this when you are just trying to do/add something fun into your life, but if you want this fun thing to be a part of your life more long-term then it is worth a little proactive, pro-body thinking.

There is nothing more frustrating than starting something new FOR your happiness/well-being and then having your back 'go out' or intense heel pain out of nowhere in the process. I want to help you avoid these fun-busters if possible. So, remember to stretch more, if you are DOING more (or are in prolonged positions more). Remember to use the 'set' position for good posture as much as you can. Remember to use counter-movements such as gentle back extension, if you are sitting/bending more. Remember to use your lower abs to help protect your lower back (and alignment down the chain). Oh, and remember to hydrate!! Also, remember that gradual is always better when it comes to avoiding negative body reactions to new activities.

Ok, now let's take integration to the next level. We will get into this more in Chapter 9, but... remember the part where you are intermittently 'dreaming up' your single-event Bucket List? Well, if any of your list involves your fitness level (a big hike, run/walk race situation, walking all over Europe, etc.), then you can also start thinking about how to integrate 'training' for these things, well in advance. If you want to walk Hadrian's Wall in England (73 miles), the Camino de Santiago de Compostela in France/Spain (480 miles), or all or parts of the Pacific Crest Trail (um, 2653 miles), or anything of significant fitness level, you can start thinking about a very gradual increase in your baseline fitness routines WAY before you plan to do it. Even if you are just planning to do something fun that will involve a lot of walking in a short period of time, it is worth thinking about ahead of time. Not just for your body-health's sake, but also so you can actually enjoy the trip/excursion.

By the way, I certainly am NOT suggesting anything like the examples I mentioned (intense stuff) need to be anywhere near your bucket list. But, I do know some people WILL do it because they really want to, no matter what the body consequences are. At the very least, I hope you think the 'training' part and planning part through as much as possible and as far ahead as possible to make it a thoroughly enjoyable experience. 2 cents!

Before I send you off to Chapter 9, here are some friendly reminders as you start your new daily-life bucket list habits!

Tips:

1) Purge what makes sense to make some 'room'
2) Gradual (for body) and consistent (for habit formation)
3) Integrate 'set' position and postural habits early
4) Integrate lower abs into the mix
5) Integrate stretching and counter-movement techniques as they apply
6) While you are integrating the daily-life habits, allow your Big-Dream Bucket List items to start flexing their muscles a bit!

Oh and...

7) Go celebrate your new baseline daily-life bucket list!!

CHAPTER 9

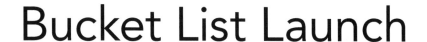

Bucket List Launch

Carpe Diem. A Latin phrase, first used by the Roman poet Horace, in 23 B.C. So, it has certainly been around for a while! It actually translates 'pluck the day,' but the sentiment of 'seize the day' is what we think of when we hear it today. I think it's interesting that those 2 words have traveled through time in a way that most people all over the world understand it and relate to it. I don't know how young I was when I first heard it, but I do know it stuck hard!

So, in the spirit of those 2 words... we officially enter the Big-Dream Bucket List chapter! I have been patiently/not-so-patiently waiting for this one! It gets me excited. I love thinking about this stuff. Not just for me, but for all of you. In fact, more so for all of you, because I have jumped on mine hard and I hope somehow this all inspires you/reminds you to get on it! Don't let time slip away. I am not saying you are, I am just saying... don't wait if you don't have to!

What I realized recently was that this is something I am incredibly passionate about. I was always personally passionate about my own life-is-short list. But, what I realized is that I am just as passionate about helping other people live out theirs. This may not sound like a huge light bulb to you, but it actually IS for me! I knew I could, and wanted to, help people body-wise with their health-fitness goals. But, ultimately, I want to help people with their body AND bucket list goals. So, here we are!

I am so curious to know your Top 3 Bucket List items. These are the single-event style ones. We have already established your daily-life bucket list items, and I hope you are devising a plan to get those guys in your daily life already. But, what we are looking at now are your once-in-a-lifetime type goals. The top 3 things you want to do or experience before you die. I mean, damn, these are big-deal things! I find it very interesting to know what other people dream of doing. In fact, you know what, you should send them to me! I will include an e-mail at the end of the book specifically for those of you who feel like sharing. I would love to know!

Ok, let's get to the extra-fun part! This is where you get to allow yourself to dream big (or small), whatever constitutes your top 3 things. I say 'or small' because your list is exactly that. Yours. It does not need to be traveling far away or doing heart-pumping things. If they are important to you, then they are big for you. I just want to be sure that you know that it could be anything, any size, anything big-deal to you.

If, like me, you have already done your (original) top 3, then awesome! I think in terms of Top-Next at this point, so I generally have a Top 1! If that's your situation, then that works, too! But, let's say you haven't been on the bucket list DOING train already. Or, you have a list, but you haven't thought about it sincerely since your 20s. Well, now is the time to revamp it! Maybe what you wanted to do in your 20s does not even apply to what your list would look like today. Change is completely allowed!! Nothing says you have to keep your old list. Now is now. Think about your old list and your current list (maybe they are the same or maybe not). Integrate and/or rewrite it completely. Whatever makes it true and current to you. I want to give you a little space to do it here...

Big-Dream Bucket List Top 3:

#1. _____

#2. _____

#3. _____

A few, I think obvious, things here. You can always change it. You can always change your order of 'importance.' BUT, ideally, when you do write them, write in order of importance and write them with intention. Of course, there is nothing magic about having 3. You could have a longer list. And, you could have only 1. But, let's shoot for 3... and then put major focus on #1!

This should feel like the best to-do list ever! It certainly should NOT make you feel stressed or inadequate. Much like the body goals you established you wanted in Part II, this isn't about what you HAVEN'T achieved or feel bad about. This is purely about figuring out what you want, and then making a decision and plan to go after it. Attitude is everything. If it is something you truly want to do, you just have to:

1) **Get your brain on board**
2) **Get your body on board**
3) **Make a REAL decision and a REAL plan to make it happen**

We have covered 1 and 2 pretty well so far, so let's tackle 3. Here's the great part. You already know all the elements of planning and deciding. AND, you have the added bonus of your

Bucket List being something you REALLY want to do, so lack of motivation is not a hindrance. So, we should look at what maybe IS hindering you. Time? Money? Courage?

Let's tackle time first. Time is actually ON your side for taking action when you think about it. Because, well, it is limited! That, by itself, puts action in your favor. I know, you meant FINDING the time is the hindrance. Yes, I get that. But, just like purging and creating time for your daily-life habits… it is there. You just have to decide it is a priority. I am not saying it is easy, I am just saying it is there. You may need to purge, rearrange, or systematically create the space in your life, but it is there if you choose to find it.

Money. Yes, this can be tricky. For some, it actually isn't a true issue, it's just a matter of priority. But for many, it is a major issue. What I can say is that money tends to live in the same realm as time in a way. Maybe you have to save for 8 years like I did. Maybe you have to rearrange and purge. Maybe you do have the resources, you just haven't decided to make it happen. Well, that's the thing with decisions. Once you DO decide, it also means IT'S ON! You will purge, rearrange, and CREATE the opportunity for yourself. You may be surprised at just how persuasive a real decision, once made, can be on you, your life, and your surroundings. Remember all those amazing things your brain can do for you once you put your mind to it'? Your brain will assist you, help you move actively (even if baby steps) TOWARDS it. You may even discover that people or opportunities will also appear and help you get there. You just need to produce the activation energy AND the net external force to get it all rolling!

Ok, let's do this. It's Go-Time! **Choose your #1 Bucket List**

item. We want to use your brain habits and all the concepts from Part I to get your brain on board with this awesome thing! **So, Step 1: Get your brain on board.** You want your thought patterns supporting you. You want your subconscious supporting you. You want your brain working FOR you towards the goal. You can even use your visualization habit directly ON your goal. You can use your already-established habit of 1-2 minutes of visualization to picture exactly what it 'looks' like and what it 'feels' like to be carrying out that dream. In sum, brain on board!

Step 2: Get your body on board. If your #1 bucket list item involves a certain level of fitness, then start thinking about how you can integrate a gradual increase in your workout plan that moves you towards conditioning for that level. Remember, as long as you are making steps towards the goal, you are in the process of making it happen. The more you DO actively, even if very small, in the direction of making it happen, the closer you get. It becomes part of a bigger plan, while incorporating it with your workouts and body habits that you have already established. Integration is helpful! Plus, it keeps you motivated and focused.

Step 3: Make a REAL decision and a REAL plan. For me, these two go together pretty much simultaneously in a lot of cases. But, honestly, when it comes to something like your #1-thing-to-do-before-you-die scenario, the decision itself comes first. It drives and creates the plan. But, for those of you who do better with a plan in order to give you the courage to decide, let's start here!

Planning is work and fun all mixed together. Let's use a trip as our example. Don't wait for the exact date to be decided - get the travel book NOW. It's an interesting thing for me that I realized years later, after many big trips in my life. The moment I bought the travel book, I knew I was going.

There has not been a single time I have purchased the book and then didn't make it happen. I am not saying that's amazing in terms of me personally, I just realized years later that for me, that was my decision moment solidified. I may not have known exactly when I was going, but I knew I was going.

Once you have the travel book, you start to see real information and real visuals towards making it happen. You are taking steps towards the outcome. If you don't take any action towards it, then you are pretty much guaranteeing it isn't going to happen. Why wait? You can take steps, even if the date isn't for years. At least you are moving towards it, not standing still.

Use all your techniques for taking small (or big) steps forward. Use Mel's 5-4-3-2-1-Go to drive to the bookstore (or click on Amazon), whatever feels better to you. Buy a map. Print some info online. Don't just read online. I say that because the more REAL it is in front of you, the bigger the step. Start making a file of information/pictures/thoughts about the trip. You are information gathering. You are putting thoughts/visuals, etc. in your brain. These can help you get there.

Think about time of year you want to be there. Or, if an event, start looking at a calendar in earnest for what your choices are, when it happens, what your options are. You are creating your own momentum when you start taking action, even if you are just getting information. Your brain is paying attention!

You can use the help of habit that you learned in Part I and II to assist you. You can create a 'travel planning' moment in your schedule. Maybe this is only 5 minutes/week or 30 min/month, but it is devoted to movement towards your dream. I know it sounds weird, but put it on your schedule. Buy a calendar if you don't have one. There is still something more effective about seeing it in front of you, on paper. Use the visualization habit ON the trip, as described, and picture the details. Picture the time of year. Picture what shoes you are taking. Yep - details, people! I know this might sound kind of over-the-top, but if you are having any trouble making things happen, all of these things add up in your brain to help make it a reality. For some, all it will take is the one step of buying the book. And, momentum and planning will take off from there. But the truth is, this doesn't happen for most people. It gets lost on a shelf, and your brain forgets it's even there. That's the one-step-and-stall effect. We want momentum instead!

Let's remember a few things about planning/deciding. Contingency plans and excuse-busters need to be at full strength! Do you remember the game King of the Mountain (or Hill, or Castle)? I loved that game as a kid. I used to play it with all the neighborhood kids after school. I was little compared to most of them, but somehow, I was very good at it. There was a neighborhood 'bully' who wasn't very happy about my skills, but I have to say, it did earn me some respect in kid-ville at the time.

Sorry, if you aren't familiar, it is just a game where 1 kid stands at the top of a hill while 1-by-1 a competitor tries to get you ... well, off the hill. In our case, it was just a small hill in someone's yard and the result would be tumbling/rolling down if you were dethroned. I do realize this probably is not suitable in a lot of scenarios today when it comes to physical games and potential injury, but this was our game almost every day for a while.

You may wonder why I am telling you about this. Contingency planning and excuse-busting makes me think of King of the Mountain. See, since I was much smaller than most of my competitors, I had to pay attention to their tendencies and 'moves' that they made. Once I picked up on those things, I could find a way to use that against them, or shut it down. Plan your moves based on not just your strength and know-how, but take into account your possible competitors' (obstacles, excuses) tendencies. You know yourself, so you have a big advantage here! Anticipate your excuse tendencies. Anticipate your obstacles. Do this ahead of time. Be ready to combat them even before they show themselves! If you anticipate them and have strategies to defeat them, you are less likely to get… dethroned … or thrown off your game.

Think about work obstacles, time obstacles, people obstacles, money obstacles, and yes, courage-competitors like fear and self-doubt. Be ready to push through these last 2. You already know they are just part of the game. You don't need any real technique for those 2. Just the courage to act anyway. Start training that habit now. The habit to act in the face of fear and/or self-doubt. These 2 competitors feed into excuse strength, so be ready for them hiding in all the excuses and obstacles to come.

Ok, before we get to our official Bucket List Launch Party, I want to give you some ideas/strategies for integrating body habits/workouts DURING your big-life activities, if it makes sense to do so. This would apply to scenarios where you maybe take an extended journey/trip somewhere and want to keep, or at least maintain, your fitness/strength level during this time. If your event is a short period of time, or is specifically fitness-related, you would not necessarily need this part. But, for those that do, there are a few things that are helpful to think about in your planning phase. Plus, it is nice to incorporate this into your life, in other travel or life-transition scenarios or extended trips.

First of all, resistance bands are glorious. They take up virtually no space in a suitcase or backpack. Resistance bands, combined with a body weight/floor routine, can be perfect for these scenarios. That's one option overall.

Another technique I have used over the years when it comes to travel workouts is something a little… different. For me, I like to work a few of the bigger muscle groups (like the ones I use gym equipment for) a little differently. Let me give you an example. Lats. Latissimus Dorsi for those that like muscle names! It is Latin for 'broadest [muscle] of the back.' In terms of strengthening, think 'lat pull-downs' or a pull-up bar. At home I use a pull-up bar. At a gym, I use the machine that has a bar overhead that you pull down towards your chest.

Let's say you don't have a bar, or a machine, or even a resistance band with you. Here's the interesting part. You technically don't need anything to make a muscle work. You just need your brain to tell it to work 'as if' it was doing the work of pulling that bar down or pulling yourself up like a pull-up action. I discovered just how effective this can be (although it sure looks weird if someone saw you doing an invisible pull-up). Oh, wait, ok, you won't actually be levitating up and down in the air (that's another book). What I mean is, you could just stand (or sit) and reach overhead for the invisible bar and use your brain to tell your muscles that you need enough force (as if you were pulling down on the overhead bar, with resistance, towards your chest). Yep. It works. I did a personal experiment using this brain-to-muscle strengthening technique for 3 months (and then again for almost a year) while I was traveling/ nomadic. Granted, I only used it for a few muscle groups that I decided to experiment on, but it worked. Weird stuff! Just sayin' … the body (and the brain) are amazing things when it comes to strengthening.

Note to body: only do what feels 'safe' in terms of stress on the muscle, no matter what technique you use. I say this because you could even strain a muscle using an invisible weight. Uh huh. I know, that would feel like a dumb injury. So even if you are creating the 'as if' force just by your brain telling your muscle to contract intensely, you still want to be aware of doing this to fatigue, not strain.

No matter what techniques (weird or not weird) you use, I recommend having a pre-planned workout routine that is your go-to travel routine. It can just be a modified version of what you do at home/gym. But, if you establish one that works for you ahead of time, using no gym/weights, then you get rid of that excuse right away. And, you can just use it in whatever scenarios you choose. You may go on a trip and decide ahead of time it is a no-workout trip. Great! Enjoy your time off! Knowing you will get right back on schedule when you return. Or, you may decide you want to keep your body exercising amidst the fun/chaos so that you keep some routine, even if much modified. Great! Also a good plan. Either way, it is a decision you make. So, you either celebrate it as a reward, or you already have a plan in place you can use and don't have to worry about 'lost ground' in the process.

It is worth noting here also that if you are still in the habit-formation stages, you may want to consider the not-too-much-time-off option. It is harder to reestablish a routine while it is still in 'stick' and 'stay' stages than it is if you have been doing it a long time. Plus, if you are in the gradually-build-a-foundation part of things, your body will appreciate the less stop-and-go versions as well. But, again, all choices that you can make depending on the situation. Just mentally establish your re-start date if you stop for a while. A big part of all of this is being in control. Have a plan. Stick to it. Or at least give yourself the option of a plan to stick to! Even if the plan is to take a break.

I hope the ideas in here can help you integrate, build, maintain, AND find balance between your brain, your body, and your bucket list! I think that is really the key. Finding the balance that works best for you, and making sure to create a foundation for yourself that you can use throughout all the big and small changes in your life. You want to be able to take care of yourself as you age, give yourself the best foundation no matter what comes at you, AND make sure to celebrate and reward yourself throughout the journey. It's about the practical (habits) and the passion (bucket list). Finding a balance and a way for them to grow together, feeding both your health/fitness AND your life-is-short-ness.

I truly do feel that the 40s are the perfect time to thoroughly re-evaluate, re-set, and re-boot. I hope this book helps you create a solid foundation that will serve you for the rest of your life. And for those of you in another decade of life, don't feel left out... this can still all apply to you, too! By taking an honest look at yourself and your life, you can then take knowledgeable action to move with intention and direction towards your goals/happiness. A thorough and realistic plan + an earnest decision = positive change. And hey, we each have a time limit, so I say ACTIVATE!

Ok, we have arrived! It's your Bucket List Launch Party!! It's official Go-Time… it's decision time. I love this moment. Know it. Feel it. Get after it and make it happen. And… cheers and a big hug, from my bucket list to yours!

The Mullen Method

Module 1:

1) Take Mental Inventory (current thought pattern lists, positive and negative)
2) Be your own Brain Boss (identify 5 pos and neg and prepare to transform them)
3) Reconnect with True-You (list 3 things you enjoyed as a kid, 3 things today)

Module 2:

1) Transform old thought patterns to new beneficial patterns (purge and replace)
2) Rep your brain and use mental fortification tools to help you re-set
3) Set baseline patterns

Module 3:

1) Set mental foundation (brain freeze, visualization, dream-wake)
2) Sustainable/excuse-busting plan
3) Take brain habit action (daily routine in motion)

Module 4:

1) Take body habit inventory (pay attention to body input habits)
2) Body mechanics baseline (identify current positions/ movement pattern and list percentages)
3) Abdominal awareness (TA engagement)

Module 5:

1) Postural corrections and 'set' positions
2) Habit-change tools and techniques to integrate corrective positions and countermeasures
3) 10 daily body habits in action (daily body baseline routine in motion)

Module 6:

1) Brain and body on board for new body/fitness goals
2) Long-term planning for workout/fitness routines
3) Integrating posture/mechanics into new goal and taking action

Module 7:

1) Finding your happy-factors (list your top 3 daily-life bucket list items)
2) Making room/time/purging in preparation
3) Activation energy tools

Module 8:

1) Re-set button (evaluate priorities and life changes)
2) Use habit progression towards your happiness (5 min mindset)
3) Integrate brain and body habits with new daily-life bucket list action

Module 9:

1) Big-Dream bucket list (list top 3)
2) Real planning (take steps towards your goal, even if small)
3) Integrate brain, body, and carpe diem attitude to make your bucket list a reality

About The Author

Diane Mullen is a licensed Physical Therapist, who earned her Master's Degree in Physical Therapy from Washington University in St. Louis in 2000. Diane earned her Bachelor of Science Degree from Purdue University in 1998, with a minor in Psychology. She worked in an orthopedic hospital-based clinic for 5 years before continuing in the profession as a traveling PT. She worked in multiple states over the next 7 years, treating people with a broad spectrum of orthopedic conditions while still managing to travel both domestically and abroad between contracts. She then worked in Seattle, WA for the next 5 years before making the decision to take some time off to travel and make some life and health changes of her own. She settled in Carlsbad, California in 2019 and embarked on a new career path, combining her knowledge and experience to create programs to address health and well-being for women their 40's.

Diane has interspersed her *life-is-short adventures* with a career in healing others. Helping others while still pursuing her own dreams and overcoming her own health obstacles along the way has been a challenge and a priority. She has always had a keen interest in the brain, decision-making, habits, and how habits assist or inhibit us from reaching our fitness and life goals.

She is the author of 43 YEAR OLD FEMALE and she is currently developing retreats for women in their 40s, with special small-group retreats in California wine country for women who are unmarried and kid-free.

Diane's methods can be applied to anyone, but she has a mission to help women in their 40s tackle age-specific challenges both mentally and physically to make their 40s their best decade yet and provide a solid foundation for the years and life-changes to come.

Diane lives in Carlsbad, California with her two drum kits and three succulents. She makes it a priority to walk to the beach every day, for what she calls wave-sound therapy.

Contact Information

Website: themullenmethod.com

Please contact Diane Mullen at:

E-mail: themullenmethod@gmail.com

As promised, an e-mail address specifically for your bucket lists! Do share! 43yearoldfemale@gmail.com

Diane mentors women in their 40's in The Mullen Method in select, small-group online programs, as well as 1-1 programs. Reservation required as space is limited.

For retreats, please contact her at themullenmethod@gmail.com with 'retreat' in the subject line. Retreat spaces are very limited. Please check website for upcoming schedules.

Charitable Contributions

Diane plans to donate a percentage of the proceeds from this book to the following 3 charities:

- Pacific Marine Mammal Center - Pacificmmc.org
- Kyani Caring Hands - Caringhands.kyani.net
- League of Women Voters - Lwv.org

Printed in the United States
By Bookmasters